100 Questions & Answers About Colorectal Cancer

Second Edition

David S. Bub, MD
Assistant Professor of Surgery
Mount Sinai School of Medicine
New York, NY

Susannah Rose, MSSW
Harvard University
Cambridge, MA

W. Douglas Wong, MD
Memorial Sloan-Kettering Cancer Center
New York, NY

JONES AND BARTLETT PUBLISHERS
Sudbury, Massachusetts
BOSTON TORONTO LONDON SINGAPORE

World Headquarters
Jones and Bartlett Publishers
40 Tall Pine Drive
Sudbury, MA 01776
978-443-5000
info@jbpub.com
www.jbpub.com

Jones and Bartlett Publishers
Canada
6339 Ormindale Way
Mississauga, Ontario L5V 1J2
CANADA

Jones and Bartlett Publishers
International
Barb House, Barb Mews
London W6 7PA
UK

Jones and Bartlett's books and products are available through most bookstores and online booksellers. To contact Jones and Bartlett Publishers directly, call 800-832-0034, fax 978-443-8000, or visit our website, www.jbpub.com.

Substantial discounts on bulk quantities of Jones and Bartlett's publications are available to corporations, professional associations, and other qualified organizations. For details and specific discount information, contact the special sales department at Jones and Bartlett via the above contact information or send an email to specialsales@jbpub.com.

The authors, editor, and publisher have made every effort to provide accurate information. However, they are not responsible for errors, omissions, or for any outcomes related to the use of the contents of this book and take no responsibility for the use of the products and procedures described. Treatments and side effects described in this book may not be applicable to all people; likewise, some people may require a dose or experience a side effect that is not described herein. Drugs and medical devices are discussed that may have limited availability controlled by the Food and Drug Administration (FDA) for use only in a research study or clinical trial. Research, clinical practice, and government regulations often change the accepted standard in this field. When consideration is being given to use of any drug in the clinical setting, the health care provider or reader is responsible for determining FDA status of the drug, reading the package insert, and reviewing prescribing information for the most up-to-date recommendations on dose, precautions, and contraindications, and determining the appropriate usage for the product. This is especially important in the case of drugs that are new or seldom used.

The authors, editor and publisher of this publication have reviewed and accepted editorial changes provided by sanofi-aventis, Inc.

Production Credits
Executive Publisher: Chris Davis
Associate Editor: Kathy Richardson
Production Director: Amy Rose
Production Editor: Daniel Stone
Associate Marketing Manager: Rebecca Wasley
Manufacturing and Inventory Coordinator: Therese Connell
Composition: Appingo
Cover Design: Jon Ayotte
Printing and Binding: Malloy, Inc.
Cover Printing: Malloy, Inc.

Library of Congress Cataloging-in-Publication Data
Bub, David S.
100 questions & answers about colorectal cancer / David S. Bub, Susannah Rose, W. Douglas Wong. -- 2nd ed.
p. cm.
Includes bibliographical references and index.
ISBN-13: 978-0-7637-5441-9
ISBN-10: 0-7637-5441-2
1. Colon (Anatomy)--Cancer--Popular works. 2. Rectum--Cancer--Popular works. I. Rose, Susannah. II. Wong, W. Douglas. III. Title. IV. Title: One hundred questions and answers about colorectal cancer.
RC280.C6B83 2008
616.99'4347--dc22

2007023320

6048

Printed in the United States of America
11 10 09 08 07 10 9 8 7 6 5 4 3 2 1

CONTENTS

INTRODUCTION

Why should we talk about colorectal cancer?

We are exposed to stories about colorectal cancer all the time. We hear about prominent celebrities and athletes diagnosed with colorectal cancer. On the news, we hear about advances in surgical approaches and new chemotherapy developments. We have friends and family who may have colonic polyps or colon cancer. Colorectal cancer is a common disease; in the year 2007, there will be an estimated 153,760 new cases of colorectal cancer diagnosed in America. It is the most common cancer involving the gastrointestinal tract in the United States, it is the third most common site of cancer overall, and it accounts for the second highest number of cancer deaths. Only lung and prostate cancer are more common in men, and only breast and lung cancer are more common in women. Although the number of new cases each year varies among ethnic groups, colorectal cancer affects men and women almost equally.

From these statistics, one could argue that we should talk about colorectal cancer because of its frequency alone. The main point; however, is that colorectal cancer is a preventable disease. We now know that almost all colorectal cancers develop from preexisting benign polyps or growths, and that with appropriate screening, benign polyps can be identified and removed, thereby preventing the cancer. Furthermore, existing cancers can be identified early and cured, sometimes even without surgery!

Since 1985, both the incidence and the mortality of colorectal cancer have been falling steadily. In 1986, 62% of patients diagnosed with colorectal cancer were cured, showing a marked improvement from the 46% cured in 1973 (that's almost a 50% improvement!). This is because colorectal cancer caught at an early stage has more than a 90% chance of being cured. Despite the knowledge that detection and removal of benign polyps by routine screening can prevent colorectal cancer and that a colorectal cancer detected early is very curable, less than a third of the eligible U.S. population has had the appropriate screening tests.

In the *Second Edition* of this book, we hope to answer most of the questions we hear in our clinical practice from people with colorectal cancer and their caregivers. Cancer is an intimidating disease and is not a popular topic of conversation. Add to that the aesthetic aspects of the colon and rectum—let's face it, a person's bowel function is a very intimate and uncomfortable topic with what might bluntly be called a high "yuck!" factor—it is clear why this discussion is avoided. We hope that we will be able to clear up some of the common misconceptions regarding colon cancer and explore many of the factors that play a role in surgical decision-making. Finally, we hope that reading this book will help readers cope with the life changes cancer brings and provide additional resources during the battle with this disease.

David S. Bub, MD
Susannah Rose, MSSW
W. Douglas Wong, MD

ACKNOWLEDGMENT

The authors gratefully acknowledge the hard work and contributions in the preparation of this book by Ms. Jenifer Levin, editor for the Colorectal Service at Memorial Sloan-Kettering Cancer Center. We would also like to thank Howard McCord, Jennifer McCord, and Eve Snee who reviewed portions of this book.

PART ONE

The Basics

What is the colon? How does it function?

What is the rectum? Why is it different from the colon?

What is cancer?

1. What is the colon? How does it function?

For you to gain a good understanding of what is happening in colorectal cancer, we need to begin with a basic lesson in the anatomy and functioning of the **large intestine**. The **gastrointestinal (GI) tract** contains the organs that digest the food we eat. From the mouth, food passes sequentially through the **esophagus** (the muscular tube joining the mouth and the stomach), the **stomach**, the **small intestine**, and finally, the large intestine. Each organ in this chain has a specialized function in digestion. The stomach stores food, churns it around, and begins digesting it with enzymes and concentrated hydrochloric acid. The small intestine, sometimes called the small bowel, uses its long length to absorb fats, proteins, and carbohydrates. The remaining waste enters the large intestine, which is made up of both the **colon** and the rectum. The large intestine is where water is absorbed, thereby preventing dehydration. The colon is extremely efficient in its function, and only a small percentage of the water leaves the body in feces (solid waste).

The colon is a tube-shaped organ inside the abdomen. It is about 5 feet long and stretches from the right side of the abdomen over to the left like an upside-down "U." The small bowel is attached to the colon by a structure called the **ileocecal valve** in the right lower section of the abdomen. The appendix, a worm-like appendage that might be the most familiar part of this unfamiliar organ, protrudes from the colon at the ileocecal junction. Beginning on the right side, contents from the small intestine move sequentially through the five sections of the large intestine, from (1) the right colon to (2) the transverse colon, (3) the descending colon, (4) the **sigmoid colon** (the "S"-shaped loop of the colon before the rectum), and finally to (5) the rectum (Figure 1). The blood supply to the colon originates from the **aorta**, the major blood vessel that brings blood out of the heart. Large blood vessels called **mesenteric vessels** arise from the aorta and fan out to create an array of smaller vessels that supply blood to the small

Large intestine
The final organ in the gastrointestinal tract. Its role is the absorption of water and nutrients from digested waste.

Gastrointestinal (GI) tract
Group of organs involved in the digestion and absorption of the food we eat.

Esophagus
Muscular tube joining the mouth and stomach.

Stomach
The sac-shaped digestive organ that is located in the upper abdomen, under the ribs.

Small intestine
Tubular organ between the stomach and the large intestine.

Colon
Part of the large intestine beginning at the cecum and continuing until the end of the sigmoid colon where the rectum begins.

Ileocecal valve
Junction of the small and large intestine.

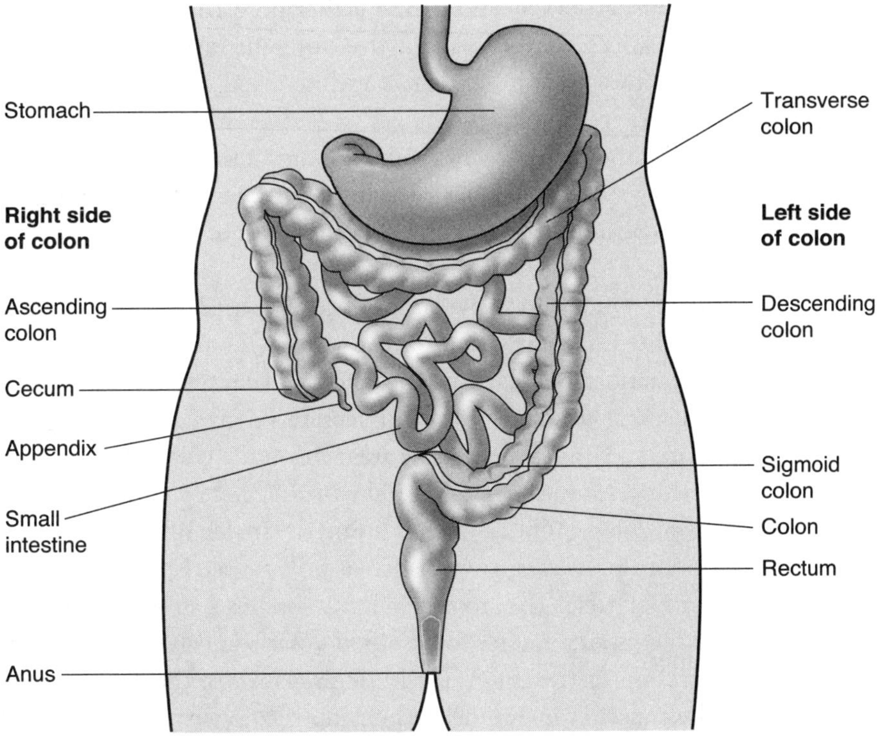

Figure 1 Anatomy of the colon. From the National Cancer Institute.

and large intestines. Because there are many interconnections among these vessels, blood flow can still be adequate even if one of the vessels becomes blocked or is removed during surgery. Within the fat (the **mesentery**) around these vessels are the **lymph nodes** that drain the colon; these lymph nodes are part of your immune system and can be quite important in combating colon cancer (see Question 7).

At this point you may wonder where this anatomy lesson is heading; isn't it enough to know there's a **tumor** in the colon and it needs to be removed? The answer is simple: colon cancer is characterized by its location within the colon, and the surgery required for its removal differs depending on the segment of colon involved. You won't know what type of surgery will be required (or the likelihood of success, or the possible aftereffects of surgery) until you know where the cancer has

sigmoid colon
The "S"-shaped loop of colon before the rectum.

Mesenteric vessels
The blood vessels that supply the large and small intestine. The lymph channels that drain the colon and rectum are adjacent to these vessels.

Mesentery
The fatty tissue surrounding the blood vessels that supply the bowel.

occurred (see Question 36). Furthermore, the extent to which the cancer has penetrated the different layers of the colon can affect the outcome of your illness and the possibility of a second episode of this cancer (called a recurrence). Thus, it is very important for you to understand these details if you're to manage your health over the long term. So with that in mind, let's continue our exploration of the colon.

The colon has four layers: (1) the **mucosa,** (2) the **submucosa,** (3) the **muscularis,** and (4) the **serosa** (Figure 2). The mucosa is the innermost layer of the colon and contains the glandular cells that absorb water and secrete mucus into the lumen, which is simply the hollow area within the colon. The mucosa is shiny, smooth, and moist, like the inside of your mouth. It is from these millions of cells lining the inside of the colon that abnormal tissue growths such as **polyps** (see Question 5) and tumors arise. The fibrous submucosa lies below the mucosa and contains microscopic blood vessels and lymph channels that supply the colon. The muscular layers of the colon (called the muscularis) are next; their job is to push the contents of the colon toward the rectum. Finally, the outermost layer of tissue is called the serosa.

Lymph nodes

Small pea-like structures that strain the interstitial fluid of bacteria, toxins, and cancer.

Tumor

Abnormal growth of tissue.

Mucosa

The moist membrane lining the inside of the colon containing small glands that secrete mucus.

Submucosa

The layer of the bowel wall between the glandular lining (mucosa) and the muscle layer.

Muscularis

The muscle layer of the bowel wall.

Serosa

Thin external lining of the bowel surface.

Polyp

Abnormal mucosal growth.

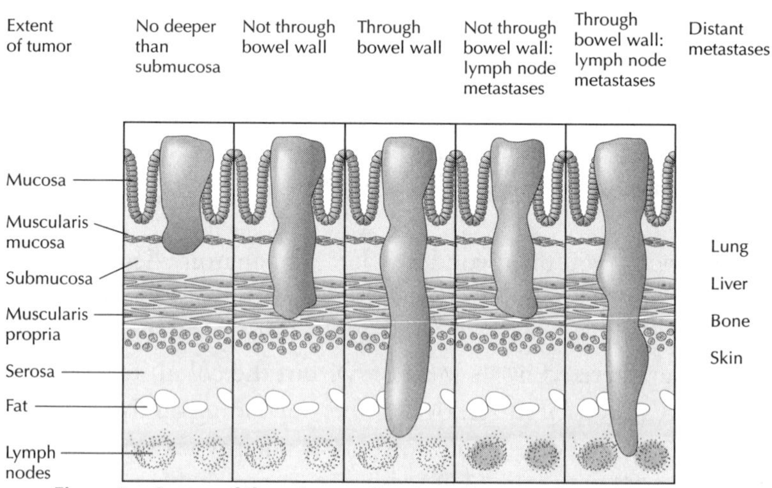

Figure 2 Layers of the colon, noting tumor penetration.

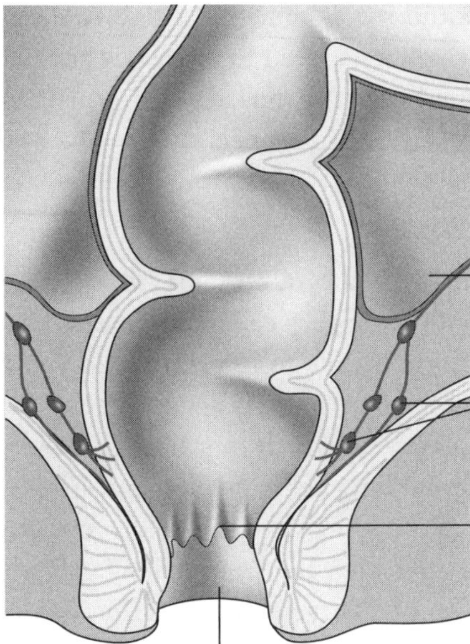

Figure 3 Anatomy of the rectum.

2. What is the rectum? Why is it different from the colon?

In the last 15 centimeters of the large intestine, the muscular bands of the colon splay out and create a pouch called the **rectum** (Figure 3). Although the main function of the colon is the reabsorption of water, the rectum functions as a reservoir designed to expand and hold stool before **defecation**. It empties through the opening called the anal canal. In the anal canal, the muscular layers of the rectum thicken into a circular band of tissue called the **anal sphincter**. The muscles of the anal sphincter, in combination with the rectal reservoir, maintain fecal continence so that defecation (the moving of one's bowels) can be put off to an appropriate time. Although the anal canal is only about 2 or 3 centimeters long, the muscles in it are crucial to our ability to perform our daily activities.

Rectum

Pouch-like structure within the lower part of the large intestine that stores fecal waste before defecation.

Defecation

The act of moving one's bowels.

Anal sphincter

Muscular band that allows us to maintain fecal continence.

Additionally, a complex group of nerves provides constant sensory input from the rectum, helping us tell the difference between gas, liquid stool, and solid stool. Reflexes from the rectum indicate when we need to move our bowels, and these reflexes, combined with the muscles of the anal sphincter, are necessary to prevent incontinence.

3. What is cancer?

Cell
The smallest structural unit of a living organism.

As you are probably aware, our bodies are composed of many different kinds of cells. Every **cell** in our bodies has its specific function, and normal cells follow regulated growth phases, have a limited life span, and stay within the boundaries of the organ or structure to which they belong—that is, you will never find a normal lung cell anywhere but in the lungs, or a cell belonging to the mucosa of the colon in the submucosa, because normal cells stay where they belong. All cells also have a normal life span or cell cycle in which they grow, reproduce (by dividing), and eventually die.

Cancer
The disordered and uncontrolled growth of cells.

Metastases
The distant spread of a cancer from its organ of origin.

Cancer is the name we give to a condition where some cells fail to follow their cell cycle rules (see Question 4). The cells become immortal and grow without limits, and they invade other structures—in some cases they even penetrate local lymph channels and blood vessels, which allows them to spread to distant organs. The cells develop distant nests of cancer in these organs, called **metastases**, which grow independently and without limit and can cause great damage.

Adenocarcinoma
Cancerous tumor arising from glandular cells.

Colorectal cancer originates from the glandular cells lining the mucosa. Cancerous tumors arising from glandular cells are called **adenocarcinomas**. As a tumor enlarges, it invades deeply into the colon. The tumor then spreads to the blood vessels and lymph channels located in the submucosa where tumor cells can spread to nearby lymph nodes or to distant organs. The deeper a tumor invades through the colonic wall, the higher its risk for distant spread and the worse a patient's prognosis (the predicted outcome of the disease).

4. What causes normal cells to become cancerous? How do genetic errors occur?

Every individual has 23 pairs of **chromosomes**—one set transferred from each parent—that store all of the information that determines how we look, function, and develop. Chromosomes are structures that contain the design for human development. Each chromosome includes thousands of instructions that determine traits like sex, eye color, and body characteristics. Like the written code in a computer program, crucial information is stored in **DNA (deoxyribonucleic acid)**, which is the building block of chromosomes. Every cell in our bodies depends upon this information to tell it how to grow, what its function is, and how it should respond to any particular situation.

Chromosomes
Thread-like structures inside the nucleus of the cell that contain the genetic instructions for cell function.

DNA (deoxyribonucleic acid)
The building block of chromosome.

When cells divide, the DNA in the cell must copy itself so that each new cell has the complete code. Sometimes, however, there's a mistake in the copy; such mistakes are called mutations. **Mutations** may affect the normal cell cycle in a way that makes the cell harmful or **malignant**. Malignant cells are usually recognized by the immune system and destroyed, but some go undetected. In these undetected cases, cell growth can go haywire. The cell can then become cancerous. It develops the ability to grow without normal limits, invade nearby structures, or spread to other organs.

Mutation
A genetic error.

Malignant
A tumor that can invade and spread.

Genetic errors can either be inherited from our parents or they can occur spontaneously. Hereditary genetic errors are called **germline mutations**, and new mistakes in DNA are called **sporadic mutations**.

Germline mutations
Errors in the genetic code that are transferred between family members.

Sporadic mutation
A genetic error that occurs randomly and is not an inherited flaw.

Certain substances cause genetic mistakes in DNA and induce cancer. For example, radiation from sun exposure is a main cause of skin cancer, asbestos and radon gas can cause lung cancer, and toxic chemicals such as benzene contribute to many other cancers. Such substances are **carcinogenic**, meaning that they are able to cause cancer. Carcinogens il-

Carcinogenic
Able to induce cancer.

lustrate how the environment has a role in the development of sporadic cancer.

Germline errors in DNA are passed from generation to generation and can cause the hereditary forms of cancer. A positive family history is a significant risk factor for colon cancer because similar genetic errors are passed down from parent to child.

5. *What is a colonic polyp?*

A polyp is any abnormal growth arising from a mucosal surface. Polyps are not limited to the mucosa of the colon, but, for example, they are also found on the lining of the nose, the stomach, and the small intestine. Polyps can be either sessile (flat) or pedunculated (on a stalk) (Figure 4).

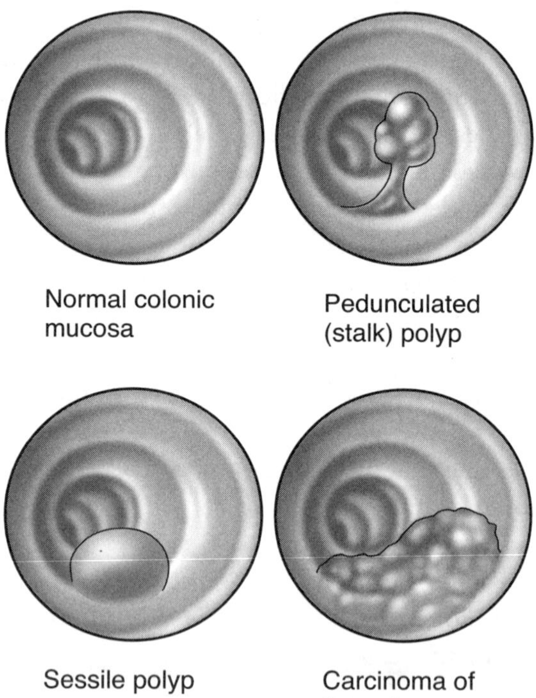

Figure 4 Neoplastic polyps: Pedunculated (stalk) and sessile.

6. Do all polyps have the same chance of containing invasive cancer?

Most polyps are **benign**, meaning that they are not cancerous. Benign colonic polyps are simply enlarged growths of tissue. Not all types of benign polyps have the potential to become cancer. Benign colonic polyps are simply enlarged growths of colonic tissue that do not have the ability to invade or spread.

Benign
A tumor that lacks the ability to invade or spread.

Adenomatous polyps, on the other hand, are neoplastic polyps, which means that they can become cancerous if they are not removed. They are made up of colonic mucosal glands and are defined by their microscopic appearance. Tubular adenomas are composed of horizontally shaped glands in the mucosa, whereas villous adenomas have fingerlike projections into the colonic **lumen**.

Adenoma
Glandular tumor arising from the mucosa of the colon.

Lumen
The area inside a hollow organ.

Adenomatous polyps are important because these are premalignant growths, meaning that over time, they grow larger and can transform into cancers. However, not all adenomas become cancerous. This progression of a benign adenoma into a malignant growth (one that can invade and spread) is called the adenoma--carcinoma sequence. Normal tissue converts into cancer in a well-defined series of events (Figure 5). This process does not take days or weeks, but rather years. In fact, when a colon cancer is identified during routine screening, it is likely that the polyp has been growing for over 10 years. During this conversion from adenoma to cancer, characteristic changes that can be seen under a microscope occur in the colon cells.

Early changes in adenomatous polyps are called dysplasia. This means that the cells are not following normal growth. When there is just a little cellular change, but in general the structure remains the same, it is called low-grade dysplasia. High-grade dysplasia indicates significant abnormalities in the cells. These abnormalities involve almost the entire muco-

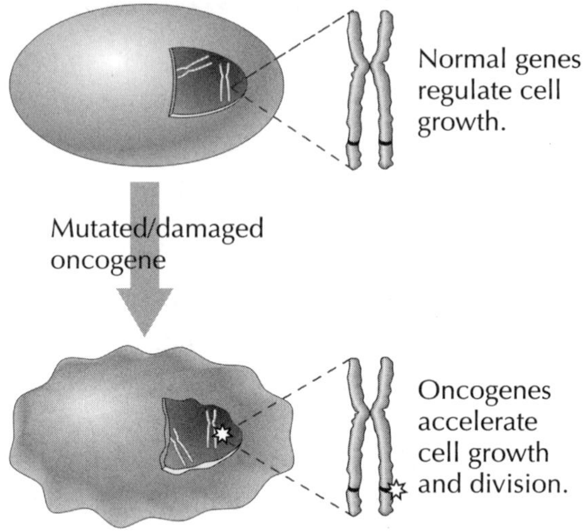

Figure 5 Normal genes and oncogenes.

sal layer of the colon. Dysplasia is the first evidence of abnormal degeneration; however, these polyps are still considered benign because they do not invade into the colonic wall and do not have the capacity to metastasize (spread beyond the bowel wall). High-grade dysplasia that is limited to the mucosal layer is called carcinoma in situ and is a form of **precancer**. Once the abnormal cells penetrate into the submucosa, the tumor becomes an invasive carcinoma, meaning that it now has the ability to spread into nearby and distant areas; it is a true cancer.

Precancer

Abnormal cells that do not yet have the capacity to spread.

Cancerous polyps can also be further characterized by **histologic** features (their microscopic characteristics), which predict tumor behavior and aggressiveness. Poor differentiation (tumors with irregular growth) and lymphovascular invasion (invasion of the lymph channels) are examples of adverse features that indicate more aggressive tumors. This information is useful to your doctor because it helps determine which sort of treatment you will need (see Question 26).

Histologic

Microscopic appearance.

The risk that a polyp contains cancer depends on its microscopic appearance and its size. The larger the polyp, the higher the risk. Also, villous adenomas have a higher chance of containing cancer than tubular polyps. Often, the way that the polyp appears to the naked eye from a **colonoscopy** (examination of the colon using a lighted instrument) helps your physician tell the nature of the polyp; however, all large polyps need to be removed for evaluation under a microscope, which is the only way to identify with certainty whether polyps are cancerous (see Question 28).

Colonoscopy
Video-endoscopy of the entire colon.

7. What are lymph nodes, and what is their relevance in colorectal cancer?

All the tissues in the body, whether in the stomach, liver, muscle, or fat, are bathed in fluid. This fluid contains absorbed nutrients and cellular waste products that are recycled through microscopic vessels, called lymph channels, back into the bloodstream to be metabolized and detoxified. Many lymph channels merge and enlarge into pea-shaped structures called lymph nodes. Lymph nodes are important because they combat infection by filtering and trapping harmful material, such as bacteria. Additionally, cancer cells can spread through these lymph channels into adjacent lymph nodes and from there into other parts of the body.

Lymph nodes drain the fluid from specific areas in the body. For example, lymph channels in the leg drain into the nodes of the groin. The lymph nodes of the colon lie within the fatty tissue surrounding their blood vessels, called the mesentery. During surgery for colon cancer, the colon and the attached mesentery are removed so the draining lymph nodes can be removed by surgery. This is important because a tumor spread to nearby lymph nodes is usually the first evidence of the spread of cancer and affects decisions about patient treatment and life expectancy. In addition, if these lymph nodes are left behind at surgery and they contain cancer cells, these cells could spark a recurrence of the original cancer.

8. Are all cancers in the large intestine the same?

Not all colorectal cancers are the same.

Not all colorectal cancers are the same. The mucosal lining of the colon absorbs water and other nutrients. Benign tumors arising from glandular cells are called adenomas, and malignant tumors are called adenocarcinomas. Adenocarcinomas are glandular tumors that grow from the mucosal lining of the colon and are the most common type of colorectal cancer. Early tumors begin as small adenomatous polyps that can turn into malignant tumors. In general, the type of cancer discussed throughout this book is adenocarcinoma. However, other rare tumors do exist and are divided into several categories.

Hormones
Chemical messengers passed through the blood stream that affect other organs.

Carcinoid tumor
Tumor consisting of neuroendocrine (hormone producing) cells.

Chemotherapy
The use of drugs to treat disease; in this case, cancerm

Stromal tumors
Rare tumor that starts in the muscular layers of the colon.

Bowel
Tumor consisting of neuroendocrine (hormone producing) cells.

Chemoradiation
Therapy consisting of chemotherapy and radiation therapy.

Neuroendocrine tumors are rare tumors of the colon. Unlike the colonic glandular cells, the function of these cells is to produce endocrine substances called **hormones**. Hormones are chemical messengers that travel through the bloodstream and affect other organs. For example, insulin is a hormone created in the pancreas that travels in the bloodstream to the liver and controls the level of blood sugar in the body. The most common type of neuroendocrine tumor, which produces a variety of different hormones, is called **carcinoid tumor**. These tumors are usually located in the appendix, small intestine, and rectum. Surgical removal of small carcinoid tumors usually cures the cancer. Poorly differentiated neuroendocrine tumors are aggressive and spread quickly to other organs, such as the lungs and liver. Patients with these tumors are treated primarily with **chemotherapy**.

Stromal tumors are rare tumors that start in the muscular layers of the colon. When discovered early, they may be benign, however, they too can transform into cancers. Because they do not arise from mucosal tissue, stromal cancers are called sarcomas. When the benign forms of this tumor are identified, surgery is recommended to prevent them from progressing into cancer. Surgery is also the mainstay of treatment for the cancerous form (sarcomas); in general, however, they are aggressive tumors with a poor prognosis.

9. Is cancer of the anal canal the same as rectal cancer?

Because the lining of the anal canal contains different cells than the colon or rectum, tumors arising in the anal canal are different from those in the colon. The anal canal contains the portion of the **bowel** that lies next to the anal sphincter muscles and is only 2 to 3 centimeters long. The treatment of anal canal tumors is different from the treatment of rectal cancers. Cancers originating in the rectum that extend into the anal canal are treated with a combination of surgery and **chemoradiation**, but anal canal tumors are often treated without surgery.

Tumors arising in the anal canal are different from those in the colon.

Squamous cell carcinoma (SCC) is the most common tumor of the anal canal. Squamous cells are flat cells that line the **epidermis** (outermost layer) of the skin. Like colonic polyps, squamous cells can grow abnormally (dysplasia) and progress into cancer. "Squamous cell atypia" is associated with papillomavirus infection (genital warts) and is therefore seen in patients with genital warts. Similarly, a higher **incidence** of SCC is seen in patients with a compromised immune system and in those with a history of **radiation therapy** to the pelvis. SCC produces symptoms similar to those of lower rectal cancer. Anal masses can cause bleeding or pain. They are often mistaken for enlarged hemorrhoids before an accurate diagnosis is made.

SCC tends to invade locally into the surrounding muscles of the anal canal and to spread to the lymph nodes in the groin. Smaller cancers arising from the skin outside the anus can be treated with local **excision** (removal). SCC used to be treated with surgery in the past. Unfortunately, this required a permanent **colostomy** (see Questions 48 and 54) and had a poor prognosis. It wasn't until the 1970s that a surgeon,

Squamous cell carcinoma (SCC)
Cancer arising from the lining of the anal canal.

Epidermis
Outermost layer of the skin.

Incidence
The number of new cases of a disease over a given time period, usually over 1 year.

Radiation therapy
The use of high-energy electromagnetic radiation to treat cancer by damaging cell DNA and causing cell death.

excision
Surgical removal.

colostomy
Stoma (a loop of bowel brought surgically out through the abdominal wall) created using the colon.

Dr. Norman Nigro, recognized that tumors of the anal canal were very responsive to a combination of radiation and chemotherapy. This regimen, the Nigro Protocol, has become the standard of care in management of these tumors. After treatment, patients require careful follow-up to make sure the tumor does not recur locally within the anal canal. We follow all of our patients closely with **endorectal ultrasound** (see Question 51) after treatment for SCC of the anal canal. Today, surgery for tumors within the anal canal is reserved for patients who fail radiation and chemotherapy or whose cancers recur. These patients require radical resections (see Question 36) and placement of a permanent colostomy (see Questions 48 and 54).

Endorectal ultrasound

radiographic test using refracted sound waves to evaluate local tumor spread within the rectum

10. Are all colorectal cancers fatal? What is my prognosis if I get colorectal cancer?

Colorectal cancer is a common disease with over 130,000 cases diagnosed each year in the United States. However, because of increased screening, the number of cancer cases is decreasing and life expectancy is increasing. So the immediate answer to the question is: No, not all colon cancers are fatal at all. In fact, more than 60% of people are cured completely (by cure or curability, we generally mean that a patient is alive and free of disease at 5 years after definitive treatment).

The most important factor in determining life expectancy is the cancer's **stage** at the time of diagnosis—that is, how far advanced it is and what effects it has had on the body (see Question 28 for more on cancer staging). When cancer is identified early, the life expectancy of patients with colorectal cancer improves. Early-stage (Stage I) tumors have an excellent prognosis, with an overall curability greater than 90%. Patients with a slightly later-stage cancer (Stage II) have a 5-year life expectancy that is greater than 80%. When the cancer spreads to local lymph nodes and is classified as Stage III, life expectancy drops to 60% to 70%. Clearly, early detection remains the key and cannot be stressed enough. Metastatic stage

Stage

A characterization of the extent of tumor growth and spread.

Early detection remains the key and cannot be stressed enough.

IV colorectal cancer can, unfortunately, rarely be cured. Some patients with limited metastatic disease are candidates for radical surgery and **adjuvant therapy** (nonsurgical treatment for cancer that helps improve long-term life expectancy; see Question 56) for potential cure; however, primary treatment is usually **palliative** (the goal is not to cure the cancer but to make the patient more comfortable), often with systemic chemotherapy (chemotherapy given **intravenously** and dispersed throughout the body). But remember: Aggressive surgical techniques and new chemotherapies continue to improve outcomes in advanced cases of colorectal cancer.

Adjuvant therapy

Nonsurgical treatment option for cancer that helps improve long-term survival.

Palliative therapy

Noncurative therapy with the aim of making the patient more comfortable.

Intravenously

Medications given through the veins.

11. Is cancer contagious?

Although genetic mutations can be passed from one generation to another, this does not mean that cancer is contagious. Cancer forms from the abnormal growth of a single individual's cells. Although genetic mutations put families at increased risk for multigenerational cases of colon cancer, cancer can never be spread by contact or exposure from one individual to another.

PART TWO

Risk and Prevention

What are the risk factors for developing colorectal cancer?

If someone in my family has colon cancer, how does that affect my risk?

Is there a gene responsible for colon cancer (a colon cancer gene)?

More . . .

12. What are the risk factors for developing colorectal cancer?

Colorectal cancer is a very common disease. In fact, the lifetime risk of developing colon cancer in the United States is about 6% of the general population. Men and women have close to an equal chance of being diagnosed with colorectal cancer. The most common risk factor is age—colorectal cancer risk increases with advancing age, peaking at age 67. The most significant risk after age is a family history of colorectal cancer. Colorectal cancer is most common among African Americans and is least common among American Indians and Hispanics.

Colon cancer, like a number of other diseases, is also related to a high-fat diet and lack of exercise. It is a striking fact that families that immigrate to the United States from regions with low overall rates of colon cancer, such as Asia, Africa, and South America, develop the same higher incidence of colon cancer commonly found in the U.S. population after only one or two generations of living here. This suggests that there is a factor in the U.S. lifestyle that elevates the risk for colon cancer and that it is not specifically related to genetic factors. Many believe that poor dietary habits in the United States account for the increased incidence of colon cancer.

Many believe that poor dietary habits in the United States account for the increased incidence of colon cancer.

You might be thinking that this information would have been a whole lot more useful had you known it before you got colon cancer. Some people even feel guilty about their diagnosis, believing that "if only I'd eaten better foods and exercised as I know I should have, I wouldn't have this problem!" The reality is, these factors are only part of the equation. There are plenty of people who eat high-fat diets and get no exercise that do not get colon cancer. There are also plenty of people who eat "right" and exercise who do get colon cancer. As discussed in Question 13, it's quite clear that this disease can be passed down in families, and perhaps you simply were not aware that your grandmother or uncle had colon cancer; you simply didn't know that you were at higher risk to start with. Ultimately, you can't ever be sure that it was your lifestyle that led to your cancer. In any case, no one ever does anything to deserve a diagnosis of colon cancer, so it's more important that you concentrate on getting rid of it than figuring out why you got it. Don't dismiss this consideration altogether, however. Remember that once your cancer is removed, the risk factors that contributed to it are still in place. So any effort you might make to alter the risks associated with your lifestyle—the only risks you can affect—will help you avoid a recurrence or a new episode of cancer (see Question 17 for more on prevention). Discuss any concerns or questions you might have with your doctor or ask that he or she refer you to a nutritionist.

13. If someone in my family has colon cancer, how does that affect my risk?

Relatives of people with colorectal cancer have a higher chance of developing cancer. The risk is two to three times higher in a person who has a first-degree relative (mother, father, sister, or brother) with colon cancer, and the closer the relation, the higher the risk will be. In other words, a person whose parent has colorectal cancer is at higher risk than a person whose brother or sister has the disease. Secondly, the risk is proportional to the number of family members with cancer. As the number of family members with colorectal cancer increases, so does an individual's risk. Finally, early age of onset is a strong risk factor.

A family history of colon cancer is an absolute indication of a need for early colonoscopic screening.

It has been proven that this risk is truly a genetic effect and not an environmental trait. A recent study compared the number of polyps in family members with the number of polyps in the patient's spouse. The risk to the spouse was equal to that in the general population, however, the risk to the family members was statistically higher because they were genetically related. A family history of colon cancer is an absolute indication of a need for early colonoscopic screening.

Kate's Comment:

When I was 13- years- old, my mother was treated for advanced colon cancer. Despite a very dismal prognosis, she survived and is in her 80s today, alive and healthy. Before my own diagnosis at 41, my grandmother, uncle, and aunt had all died of colon cancer in their 30s. My mother and a cousin had had cancer and lived. So, although I knew the disease could be fatal, Mom and Sandy were healthy, and that gave me great hope and encouragement.

Despite such an extensive family history of colon cancer, I never really realized that I could get it myself. However, after what I thought was an unusual bout of stomach flu, I went to the emergency room in pain expecting, at most, an appendectomy. Five days later, I was in surgery having a large malignant tumor removed from my **cecum**. *I don't think I even considered asking my doctor for statistical chances at the time. I just started managing life with cancer day by day. My father came to the hospital every afternoon and sat next to the bed while I got stronger. He had done the same thing for my mother, years earlier. His presence was quietly positive and helped enormously.*

Cecum

The pouch-like structure that is the first segment of the colon.

Being both realistic and positive is a difficult balance. When a new colon cancer developed 8 years later, I knew more about the statistics of survival. Still, I expected to go on living, as best as I could, as long as I could. It has been 20 years now, with no further evidence of disease.

14. Is there a gene responsible for colon cancer (a colon cancer gene)?

It can be frustrating to think that with all of the available science and technology, we do not have genetic markers that can identify patients with colorectal cancer earlier or help in the treatment of the disease. Although this is mostly true, a great deal has been learned during the past two decades regarding the genetic abnormalities associated with colorectal cancer. We have known about the familial risks for colorectal cancer, so clearly a gene, or several genes, must be involved in cancer formation. Several of these genes have been identified through extensive research and by examining families that have many cases of colorectal cancer. We have found that it is not usually only one abnormal gene, but a series of genetic mistakes that convert normal colon cells into cancerous cells.

Although the identification of these genes has been important for our understanding of the transformation of normal colon cells into cancer cells, in general they have not been useful in identifying patients who are at risk for sporadic (nonhereditary) cases of colorectal cancer—yet. However, these genes have been crucial in identifying patients who have hereditary syndromes and are at risk for colorectal cancer. Some of the identified cancer genes and the hereditary syndromes they are associated with are discussed below.

Familial Adenomatous Polyposis (FAP): FAP is an inherited syndrome in which affected individuals develop multiple polyps throughout their colon. Although the normal population may develop a few abnormal polyps in the fifth or sixth decade of life, by the time patients with FAP reach their late teens, hundreds of polyps carpet the entire colon and rectum. These polyps are adenomatous polyps and progress into cancer over time.

Familial Adenomatous Polyposis (FAP)

Disease characterized by the development of multiple adenomatous polyps throughout the colon, usually at a young age.

The gene responsible for FAP is called the adenomatous polyposis gene (or APC gene). A parent with FAP has a 50% chance of passing the syndrome on to his or her children. Mutations in the APC gene have also been found in sporadic (non-inherited) cases of colorectal cancer as well, suggesting that these mutations may be a first step in the conversion of normal colonic tissue into an adenomatous polyp.

Unfortunately, over time, all untreated patients with FAP develop colorectal cancer, so **prophylactic** surgery (surgery to prevent cancer) is usually necessary. Although there is

Prophylactic

For the purpose of prevention.

evidence that treatment with anti-inflammatory medications like **sulindac** may decrease the number of recurrent polyps in these patients, there is no definitive medical therapy for FAP, and these medications should not be used as a substitute for surgery. There is a milder form of the disease in which patients have relatively few polyps (fewer than 100) in the colon; in a few cases, patients with this milder form of FAP can undergo frequent colonoscopic screening with colonoscopy, and removal of these polyps may be an option. However, all patients with full-blown FAP and most patients with the milder form eventually need surgical resection (removal) of the entire colon and rectum to prevent the inevitable cancer formation. Total **proctocolectomy** (removal of the colon and rectum) is the current standard of care. A reconstructive procedure called the ileoanal pouch or "J" pouch operation can be performed, making a "new rectum" out of the small intestine so that a permanent stoma is not necessary (see Questions 45, 53, and 54).

Sulindac

A nonsteroidal anti-inflammatory drug that may help prevent formation of colonic polyps.

Proctocolectomy

Surgical removal of the rectum.

Sigmoidoscopic screening (see Question 20) has always been recommended for the children of parents with FAP beginning in their early teens and repeated every year. Children with many polyps are candidates for prophylactic total proctocolectomy. The development of genetic testing now allows screening to be directed at family members who are identified by a blood test to have the same mutation as the family member with the disease. First, however, the mutation must be confirmed in the blood of the family member with the disease; only then can genetic testing be reliably offered to family members to identify who is at risk of having this disease. If the genetic test results of other family members are positive, then they should undergo intensive screening because they will inevitably develop this disease. If, however, the family member's genetic test result is negative, then that person is not at risk for this disease and can wait until later in life to undergo the same risk screening that the general population undergoes. If the mutation is not identified in the affected family member, then genetic testing of other family members cannot be relied upon, and all family members should undergo intensive screening. For these reasons, we recommend that FAP families be directed to specialized centers for appropriate testing and management.

Hereditary Nonpolyposis Colon Cancer (HNPCC): During the late 60s, Dr. Henry Lynch identified families with a higher incidence of colorectal cancer and associated cancers of the stomach and uterus. Unlike FAP, however, colorectal cancer developed in only 70% to 80% of people who were suspected to have this mutation. In addition, these patients did not have thousands of polyps like those with FAP. The syndrome was named Lynch Syndrome and has since been classified as HNPCC. The colorectal **neoplasms** in HNPCC families occur at younger ages (in the 40s) and are more common in the right side of the colon. Some researchers believe that the conversion of adenomas to cancers may occur more quickly in patients with HNPCC; however, stage for stage, these tumors have a better prognosis than sporadic cancers (those not passed on genetically).

Hereditary Nonpolyposis Colon Cancer (HNPCC)

Syndrome of inherited colon cancer and other associated cancers that is not associated with the familial adenomatous polyposis syndrome.

Neoplasms

Abnormal growth of cells, a tumor.

In 1990, an international collaborative group developed research criteria to identify families who are at risk for this genetic syndrome, which would require early screening (Table 1).

Table 1 The Amsterdam criteria (3–2–1 rule)
1. Three or more relatives with histologically proven (i.e., proven through study of cells and tissue) colon or rectal cancer. One should be a first-degree relative of the other two.
2. Colorectal cancer involving two or more generations.
3. One or more cases diagnosed before age 50.

Rigorous screening with colonoscopy (see Question 20) is necessary in these families beginning at age 20. Recently, genetic markers associated with HNPCC have been identified. Several mutations have been identified; these occur on different genes, but they all ultimately affect a similar group of

DNA repair proteins. Unlike people with FAP, not everyone with HNPCC will develop colorectal cancer. Prophylactic proctocolectomy (preventive removal of the colon and rectum) is therefore not necessarily indicated, and management consists of early and frequent colonoscopic screening. Families fulfilling the **Amsterdam criteria** (screening to identify families with HNPCC) should also consider consultation at specialized institutions that have hereditary cancer registries (extensive and organized lists) and genetic counseling and testing capabilities. Ongoing screening for cancers of the ovary and **endometrium** (the lining of the uterus), as well as other associated cancers, is also required. When individuals identified with HNPCC develop colon cancer, the recommended treatment is usually total colectomy (surgical removal of the colon) because of the high risk of colon cancer formation in the future. In most cases, the rectum can be saved and a permanent stoma is not required.

Amsterdam criteria

Screening guidelines used to identify families with hereditary nonpolyposis colon cancer (HNPCC).

Endometrium

The lining inside the uterus.

Kate's Comment:

I have an unusually strong family history of colon cancer. I have had two primary malignant colon tumors, as well as breast cancer and ovarian cancer, which are related to hereditary non-polyposis colon cancer syndrome. I need to be checked every year with a colonoscopy for colon polyps or an early cancer. I have been tested for the genes that are related to HNPCC and have urged my children and my sisters to have genetic counseling and testing. If they decide not to have genetic testing or if they are found to be positive, they should have annual colonoscopies and be watched carefully for related cancers of the uterus, ovary, urinary tract, and skin.

Carrying the gene is a heavy burden. It is actually easier to cope with my own cancer than with the thought of one of my sons or one of my sisters getting cancer.

15. What is diverticulosis, and is it related to colorectal cancer?

Diverticula are pockets of colonic mucosa that penetrate small weaknesses in the colonic wall. They are common in older Americans and are thought to be caused by a low-fiber diet. Diverticula are primarily located in the sigmoid colon, the thick muscular wall of which pushes solid stool into the rectum. Diverticulosis is a benign process and is found in more than 50% of Americans over the age of 60. However, it can cause infection and bleeding.

Although diverticulitis may be mistaken for colorectal cancer, it is not a cause or risk factor for colorectal cancer.

Stool can get trapped inside one of these pockets, causing the diverticula to swell and become infected. This is called **diverticulitis.** Mild diverticulitis is treated with antibiotics and does not require hospitalization. Advanced diverticulitis, however, can cause obstruction or perforation of the colon and abscess (collection of pus) in the abdomen. Any of these symptoms can be confused with an advanced colon cancer, and surgery is often necessary just to make the exact diagnosis.

Diverticulitis
Inflammation of a diverticulum.

Although diverticulosis is a common finding on a colonoscopic screening, and although diverticulitis may be mistaken for colorectal cancer, it is not a cause or risk factor for colorectal cancer.

16. What are ulcerative colitis and Crohn's disease? Do these inflammatory bowel diseases cause colorectal cancer?

Ulcerative colitis is an inflammatory bowel disease. So is another disorder, called **Crohn's disease.** Patients with ulcerative colitis develop inflammation of the mucosa of the colon, usually in their late teens and early 20s. Symptoms include crampy abdominal pain, diarrhea with mucus, bowel urgency, and rectal bleeding. It is thought to be an autoimmune disease and is treated with immunoregulatory drugs, such as cortisone and aspirin derivatives. Ulcerative colitis

Ulcerative
Inflammatory disease affecting the mucosa of the large intestine.

Crohn's disease
An inflammatory bowel disease that can affect any part of the gastrointestinal tract.

generally develops in the rectum first and then moves up the colon, toward the beginning, until the entire colonic mucosa is affected. Inflammation is limited to the colon and does not affect the remainder of the GI tract. But patients with ulcerative colitis may develop other symptoms, including skin disorders, arthritis, and disease of the bile ducts.

Pancolitis
Colitis involving the entire colon.

Biopsy
A procedure in which tissue is removed and examined.

Occult
Hidden; not obvious to the naked eye.

Ileostomy
Stoma created with small bowel.

Restorative proctocolectomy
A surgical procedure in which the entire colon and rectum are removed, but a rectum is created using a pouch constructed from small bowel (J-pouch).

Proctoscopy
Evaluation of the rectum using a rigid or flexible endoscope.

Anal canal
the end of the gastrointestinal tract where the rectum is surrounded by the muscles of the anal sphincter.

The incidence of colon cancer is increased in patients with ulcerative colitis and may be the result of the chronic inflammation of the colon. The risk is higher in patients with **pancolitis** (colitis involving the entire colon) than in those with only left-sided disease. The risk of colorectal cancer begins about 8 to 10 years after diagnosis, and the incidence increases by about 1% with each succeeding year. Colorectal cancers that occur in patients with ulcerative colitis are often more advanced at diagnosis. Therefore, frequent screening in patients with ulcerative colitis is mandatory. Beginning 8 years after diagnosis, colonoscopy should be performed every 1 to 2 years, and multiple random **biopsy** specimens of the colon should be taken to look for dysplasia. If dysplasia is discovered by colonoscopy, prophylactic surgery is recommended.

If a cancer develops in a patient with ulcerative colitis, the entire colon needs to be removed because of the increased risk of a secondary **occult** (hidden, not obvious to the naked eye) tumor. Removal of the colon and the rectum (proctocolectomy) cures patients with ulcerative colitis. Proctocolectomy and placement of a permanent **ileostomy** (a loop of small bowel brought out surgically through the abdominal wall) eliminate the risk of cancer. As an alternative to proctocolectomy and permanent ileostomy, surgeons can perform a **restorative proctocolectomy**. During a restorative proctocolectomy, the entire colon and rectum are removed, but a "new rectum" (a neorectum) is created using a pouch of small bowel (commonly called a J-pouch). Generally, this operation reduces the risk of cancer to almost zero; however, patients may need to continue to have yearly screening with **proctoscopy** to examine the J-pouch and **anal canal**.

Crohn's disease can affect any part of the GI tract from the mouth all the way to the anus. Unlike ulcerative colitis, the inflammation seen in Crohn's disease extends through the entire thickness of the bowel wall and is characterized by strictures (narrowing of the bowel because of scarring, inflammation, or tumor) and fistulas (abnormal passage between two hollow organs).

Treatment includes immunoregulatory drugs, such as cortico-steroids and azathioprine (**Imuran**). The natural history of Crohn's disease is one of alternating flare-ups and remissions. Treatment is mainly medical, and surgery is reserved for complications such as severe strictures, abdominal infection, and symptomatic fistulas. Although the risk of developing cancer in Crohn's disease is not as well defined as is the risk in ulcerative colitis, it is believed to be higher than in the general population. For this reason, individuals with Crohn's disease of the colon require the same screening as those with ulcerative colitis. If dysplasia (microscopic finding of abnormal cell growth) is found in patients with Crohn's disease, proctocolectomy may be necessary.

Imuran
Drug that suppresses the body's immune system.

Prognosis
The predicted course of the disease.

Mortality
The death rate from a specific disorder.

17. What can I do to prevent colorectal cancer? Have any medications or vitamins been proved to reduce risk?

One of the main points we hope to make in this book is that colorectal cancer is an extremely preventable disease, and it has an excellent **prognosis** when it is identified and treated early. We divide preventive measures into categories. Primary prevention aims to reduce the risk of initially developing colon cancer. Secondary prevention consists of measures like routine screening, which reduce cancer **mortality** and increase life expectancy.

Colorectal cancer is an extremely preventable disease.

Primary colorectal cancer prevention is uncomplicated and common sense. Altering harmful lifestyle habits is very important to cancer prevention (see Question 12). Poor diet, lack

Altering harmful lifestyle habits is very important to cancer prevention.

of exercise, and smoking all have been associated with higher rates of colon cancer. By simply changing these habits, you can decrease your chance of developing colorectal cancer, as well as other diseases. However, you can play an even more active role in decreasing your chance of getting colorectal cancer. It has been suggested that supplementation with vitamins and other nutrients may help in this battle. The following sections outline some of the more commonly discussed supplements and the data regarding their role in preventing cancer.

- Calcium: Some evidence suggests that calcium may help tumors from forming in the colon. When studied in animal models, calcium reduced the number of polyps formed in response to carcinogens and high-fat diets. In humans, calcium carbonate has been shown to decrease the incidence of adenoma formation. Although it has not been proved conclusively that calcium prevents colon cancer, calcium is a benign supplement that can also prevent osteoporosis, and it can be taken safely in small doses.
- Folate: Folate is a micronutrient found abundantly in fruits and vegetables. A large study of nurses who were taking supplemental folate found a decreased risk of colorectal cancer. This small benefit became evident only after many years of folate use. Folate may reduce the risk of colorectal cancer in people who have a genetic predisposition to it. It can be taken in the form of a daily multivitamin.
- Vitamins A, C, and E: Many studies have been conducted, but they have not demonstrated a significant reduction in colorectal cancer risk as a result of supplementation with these vitamins.
- Selenium: Some studies have suggested that the incidence of colorectal cancer is higher in geographic regions where selenium is deficient. This was confirmed in one multicenter, randomized research trial that showed that cancer occurred less often in people whose

diet was supplemented with selenium in the form of brewer's yeast. In high doses, however, selenium can damage the liver, so the dosage should be increased cautiously.

- **Nonsteroidal Anti-Inflammatory Drugs (NSAIDs):** Non-steroidal anti-inflammatory drugs inhibit the action of cyclooxygenase, an enzyme involved in the inflammatory process. Concentrations of cyclooxygenase have been proved to be higher in colorectal cancers, so medications that inhibit cyclooxygenase may also decrease cancer. Sulindac, an NSAID, decreased the incidence of colonic adenomas in animal models. Additionally, in small studies in which sulindac was given to patients with familial adenomatous polyposis (FAP), the number of polyps identified on follow-up **endoscopy** (procedure in which a lighted instrument is used to examine a body cavity) was decreased. Larger studies using aspirin to prevent cancer have shown that it may decrease the incidence of polyp formation in the colon. Unfortunately, the use of high doses of aspirin is associated with stomach and duodenal ulcers. However, in patients with no risk factors for ulcer disease, a baby aspirin may be beneficial. Ongoing studies are underway using both aspirin and specialized inhibitors of cyclooxygenase, such as Celebrex, that may reveal a more significant benefit in the future.

Nonsteroidal Anti-Inflammatory Drugs (NSAIDs)
Category of drugs that reduce inflammation; includes aspirin, ibuprofen, sulindac.

Endoscopy
Using a lighted instrument to look inside a body cavity.

These are the main supplements that have been investigated for the prevention of colon cancer. Other herbal medications or colonic enemas ("high colon-ics"), although touted as saviors in the battle against colon cancer, have not been demonstrated to prevent cancer.

In summary, a healthy lifestyle can go a long way in the primary prevention of colorectal cancer. By following simple dietary guidelines, drinking alcohol in moderation, following a basic exercise program, and not smoking, you can decrease your risk of developing colorectal cancer. Moderate doses of dietary supplements in the form of multivitamins, high-calcium diets, and aspirin may be beneficial.

With routine screening, colon cancer can be prevented by the removal of precancerous polyps.

Fecal occult blood testing (FOBT)

Laboratory test that examines stool for microscopic traces of blood.

The key to secondary prevention is proper screening. With routine screening, colon cancer can be prevented by the removal of precancerous polyps and, if already established, colon cancer can be diagnosed at an earlier stage, resulting in better life expectancy. For this reason, it is unacceptable that less than 30% of the eligible U.S. population undergoes colorectal cancer screening. For example, by using a simple, noninvasive test that measures the stool for hidden blood every year, the mortality from colorectal cancer dropped by one third in a study population! **Fecal occult blood testing** (**FOBT**, see Question 19) was the first screening test that demonstrated better life expectancy after colorectal cancer. Although FOBT can identify early cancers, colonoscopy can both diagnose and treat early polyps. The National Polyp Study was a national multicenter trial evaluating colonoscopy in the prevention of colon cancer. Over 9,000 patients were referred for this trial which compared colonoscopic screening for colorectal cancer with regular observation. Repeat colonoscopy in patients with colonic polyps prevented almost 90% of expected colon cancers. Regular screening has repeatedly been proven to identify more cancers at earlier stages.

PART THREE

Screening and Diagnosis

How will I know if I have colorectal cancer?

What kind of screening is available, and at what age should I start?

I was found to have blood in my stool. My doctor recommended a colonoscopy. What is that?

More . . .

18. How will I know if I have colorectal cancer?

Routine screening remains the cornerstone of early colorectal cancer diagnosis.

Like many other diseases, people with colorectal cancers do not have symptoms until the cancers are somewhat large. Unfortunately, by this time, the cancer may have spread to other organs, and cure may be impossible. Therefore, routine screening remains the cornerstone of early colorectal cancer diagnosis. As colorectal cancers grow, however, warning signs will arise, and these should prompt you to get further medical evaluation.

A change in your bowel habits is the most common symptom of colorectal cancer.

A change in your bowel habits is the most common symptom of colorectal cancer. Colorectal cancer can block the normal flow of feces and create irregular bowel function. You may notice a change in the way your stool looks, so that what once was big and bulky may now be narrow and thin. You may become constipated and need to take laxatives, something you never needed to do before. Large rectal cancers can produce sensations of rectal fullness and incomplete evacuation after defecation. More frequent and smaller bowel movements, associated with feelings of urgency, can represent loss of space in the rectum due to the presence of a large tumor. Rectal pain is not that common; however, it can be present with lower cancers that infiltrate the muscles of the anal sphincter. Finally, in the most advanced form, cancers can grow so large that they cause severe constipation, abdominal bloating, and even complete obstruction. Although many of these symptoms can be associated with normal bowel activity, if these changes persist, you should promptly seek medical attention.

Colorectal cancers can also cause blood to be mixed with the stool. For example, colorectal cancers bleed easily when they are contacted by passing stool. Most of this bleeding is small and is not noticeable in normal bowel movements. This is called "occult" bleeding and is common when tumors are located in the right side of the colon. Even though this bleeding is often too minimal to be seen, it is persistent and, over time, can cause **anemia** (a decrease in the number of circulating red blood cells). Anemia makes you feel tired or easily fatigued. Although anemia has many causes, any older person who is found to be anemic should have a screening colonoscopy to rule out colonic polyps. Bleeding from rectal cancer is usually more obvious, with bright red streaks of blood seen on the stool, toilet paper, or in the toilet bowl. This is why it is often mistaken for bleeding hemorrhoids. A doctor should evaluate any new rectal bleeding, even if you have had a past history of hemorrhoids. Finally, constitutional symptoms like abdominal distention, **jaundice** (signs of liver failure), and bone pain are associated with advanced tumors and metastatic spread. These cancers generally cannot be treated surgically.

Anemia
Decreased number of red blood cells.

Jaundice
The symptoms that are associated with liver failure; especially a yellow color to your skin and the whites of your eyes.

In summary, the main symptoms seen with colorectal cancers are a change in bowel habits, anemia, and rectal bleeding. Most people won't have any of these findings until the tumor is fairly advanced. For this reason, it is a bad idea to wait for symptoms to develop. Screening for colorectal cancer allows for identification of colorectal cancer at earlier stages, and therefore makes it more likely that the cancer can be treated successfully.

It is a bad idea to wait for symptoms to develop.

19. What kind of screening is available, and at what age should I start?

We know that colorectal cancer screening leads to earlier diagnosis of cancers and therefore improves life expectancy. The problem, however, is creating an effective screening test. From a purely medical standpoint, a successful screening test is noninvasive and inexpensive, and it accurately diagnoses occult (hidden) disease at a treatable stage. The Papanicolaou ("Pap") smear, which identifies early cervical cancer, has been one of the most successful screening tests to date. Yearly pelvic examinations detect early cervical dysplasia, allowing for surgical cure. This has markedly decreased the mortality from cervical cancer. Measuring the blood prostate-specific antigen level has resulted in earlier detection of prostate cancer.

Although the perfect test for colon cancer does not yet exist, the use of a combination of studies is extremely effective for diagnosis and is responsible for the declining rates of colon cancer.

Screening doesn't help if you don't get it.

Flexible sigmoidoscopy

A test that provides an inside look at the rectum and lower part of the colon.

Barium Enema

An x-ray examination of the colon using a contrast material to highlight the area being examined.

But screening doesn't help if you don't get it. The fact that less than 30% of the U.S. population gets adequate screening emphasizes this point and illustrates the potential survival benefits that are still possible. Colorectal cancer screening is usually initiated by your family physician and begins with a complete physical examination, including digital rectal examination and some basic blood tests. Other screening tests include fecal occult blood testing, **flexible sigmoidoscopy**, colonoscopy, and **barium enema** (see Questions 17 and 20). A barium enema is an x-ray examination of the colon. Because the walls of the colon are very thin, they do not absorb x-rays well and cannot create a good image for evaluation. Contrast material is needed to coat the bowel wall, which highlights abnormalities and makes x-ray examination easier. Two materials are commonly used. The most effective one for coating the bowel wall is barium, a thick, chalky, white material. Gastrografin is a liquid that is used occasionally instead of barium; however, it is not as effective. The barium is given as an enema that fills the entire colon, and large polyps or cancers can be seen on the x-ray. This is called a single-contrast enema. To further enhance the image so that smaller polyps and abnormalities can be seen, air can be insufflated into the colon (air is blown into the colon) after the barium; this expands the lumen and creates a double contrast. Better interpretation can be achieved with this double-contrast technique.

Although it can be an uncomfortable examination, there are few risks associated with a barium enema, and it does not require any kind of sedation. However, barium enema does require a complete bowel cleansing preparation the day before to empty the bowel of waste. It is also necessary to hold the barium inside the colon for the duration of the examination.

The barium enema is an excellent medical test, but it does have some limitations. A barium enema identifies large colonic lesions more than 80% of the time, but it recognizes small polyps less then 1 centimeter large only 50%–60% of the time. Residual stool inside the colon can complicate interpretation and make additional studies necessary. Another disadvantage is that the barium enema can be used only for diagnosis; it does not allow for therapeutic interventions. For these reasons, it has largely been replaced by colonoscopy for evaluation of the entire colon. Barium enema is used mainly when patients are unable to undergo colonoscopy.

Screening tests should be minimally invasive, easy to perform, and oversensitive. In this way, an individual who is at higher risk can be selected for additional and more accurate procedures. Fecal occult blood testing (FOBT) is an example of an inexpensive, minimally invasive, overly sensitive test for colon cancer that is used to identify patients who need further workup.

FOBT checks for microscopic evidence of blood in the stool by utilizing an enzymatic reaction with **hemoglobin**, the oxygen-carrying protein in the blood. The stool is tested for blood because colon cancers bleed more often than regular colonic mucosa. About two thirds of cancers bleed during the course of a week, usually without being noticed. Because these tumors may bleed intermittently, the more samples checked at different times, the higher the likelihood of correctly finding a positive result. Your doctor will ask you to collect three samples of stool from two different sites using a wooden stick. He will ask you to collect three samples this way. These samples will then be tested to detect blood.

Hemoglobin
Protein in the blood responsible for carrying oxygen.

FOBT is a good screening test. It is inexpensive, easy to perform, and very sensitive, meaning that it will identify over 90% of cases of large polyps or cancers. However, a large number of positive reactions can be explained by other abnormalities (false-positive result). For example, enlarged hemorrhoids, stomach ulcers, or even bleeding gums can cause a false-positive result. Therefore, FOBT, although sensitive, has limited accuracy and is used to identify patients who will require additional workup, like colonoscopy or barium enema. FOBT performed yearly, combined with flexible sigmoidoscopy every 5 years, is an effective screening regimen. However, colonoscopy is viewed by many as the most effective screening modality currently available. For average risk individuals, screening should begin at age 50 (see Question 24).

20. I was found to have blood in my stool. My doctor recommended a colonoscopy. What is that?

Patients who are at high risk for colon cancer, or those with abnormal findings on fecal occult blood testing, need further evaluation using either an **endoscope** (a lighted instrument used to look inside a body cavity) or a barium enema combined with an endoscopic exam. Colonoscopy can also be used as the primary screening examination. Colonoscopy has become the standard of care for cancer screening, and thousands are performed daily across the United States.

Endoscope

A lighted instrument used to look inside a body cavity.

Endoscopy is the use of lighted instruments to look inside a hollow organ. Originally, endoscopes were rigid and allowed only limited examination of the esophagus and rectosigmoid colon. Some of these instruments are still used frequently today. If you have rectal or anal symptoms, your doctor may still use a rigid scope called a proctoscope. This instrument is only 20 to 25 centimeters long and can identify enlarged hemorrhoids or polyps in the lower portion of the colon and the rectum. Although the procedure is uncomfortable, a rigid proctoscopy should not hurt and does not require sedation.

With the advent of fiber-optic light technology, flexible endoscopes have been developed to negotiate the twists and turns inside the colon. Visualized images are displayed on television monitors and are greatly magnified for easier evaluation. These scopes also contain special channels that allow instruments to be placed directly into the colon for biopsy or polyp removal.

A flexible sigmoidoscope is a short fiber-optic scope that can explore the lower half of the colon. It is about 60 centimeters long and about the diameter of your little finger. Flexible sigmoidoscopy is performed as an ambulatory procedure in your doctor's office. It does not require any sedation, and the entire procedure lasts only about 5 to 10 minutes. Air is insufflated (blown) into the colon, distending the bowel so that your doctor can see it adequately. The insufflated gas will give you an uncomfortable, bloated feeling, but should not be painful. During the procedure, you may feel the urge to move your bowels, or even feel as if you are moving your bowels. This is a normal sensation caused by the passing scope and injected air. Do not be embarrassed if you need to expel some air during the procedure because this is entirely normal. Flexible sigmoidoscopy can visualize the rectum and the lower half of the colon, however, the upper half of the colon is not evaluated. It is therefore possible that polyps or even cancers in the top half of the colon can be missed by flexible sigmoidoscopy. For this reason, there has been a movement toward using colonoscopy rather than sigmoidoscopy as the baseline screening examination of choice.

Colonoscopy is a more complete examination of the colon than flexible sigmoidoscopy. A colonoscope is 6 feet long and evaluates the entire colon. Because the colonoscope negotiates all the curves within the colon, including the large curves, it is more uncomfortable and requires sedation to make you more comfortable. For this reason, although flexible sigmoidoscopy can be performed in your doctor's office as an ambulatory procedure, colonoscopy is performed at specialized endoscopy units, where you will be monitored because sedation is used. Although you will remain awake during the endoscopy and can follow simple instructions (like "roll over" or "bend your legs"), you will be in a "twilight zone" and likely will not remember any part of the procedure. A standard colonoscopy lasts only about 15 to 30 minutes but can take longer in some cases. A colonoscopy can be more challenging to complete in patients who have undergone abdominal surgery or in those with long colons.

The bowel preparation needed for colonoscopy is different than that needed for sigmoidoscopy. Before undergoing flexible sigmoidoscopy, two Fleet® enemas are used 1 or 2 hours prior to the test, and no dietary changes are needed. But colonoscopy requires cleansing of the entire colon and is more involved. Preparation begins the day before by limiting the diet to liquids only. A bowel-cleansing regimen will begin in the late morning, using a bowel preparation. Several commercial preparations are available. GoLYTELY®, which is commonly prescribed, requires consumption of a gallon of liquid. It comes in a variety of flavors and is very effective in emptying the colon; however, the entire solution needs to be taken for complete results. Fleet® Phospho-soda® comes in two small portions that are taken with juice. It is generally as effective as GoLYTELY® and may be easier to tolerate. Other bowel preparations exist and can be prescribed by your physician.

All bowel preparation solutions cause rapid bowel emptying. A few hours after beginning the regimen, you can expect to go to the bathroom frequently. It is very easy to become dehydrated during preparation, so you should try to drink plenty of clear liquids over the course of the day. In addition, these cathartics (especially Fleet® Phospho-soda®) can produce electrolyte shifts in the blood and must be taken with care in patients who have kidney problems or heart disease. When your bowel movements become a transparent liquid, this indicates that you have adequately completed the preparation. Continue to drink lots of liquids during the day. You should also take your regular medications the morning of the procedure with a small drink of water (there are a few exceptions to this; see Question 21). Because you will receive sedation during your colonoscopy, a friend or family member must accompany you home after the procedure. There are no exceptions. Although you probably won't want to return to work, you will be free to return to normal activities later in the day.

21. Isn't colonoscopy risky?

Colonoscopy is a very safe procedure. However, like any medical intervention, it does carry a risk, albeit small, for complications. The major complications of colonoscopy are post-procedure bleeding and colonic perforation (piercing). Bleeding occurs in about 3 of every 1,000 colonoscopies and is much more common in patients who needed therapeutic interventions, like polyp removal or biopsy. Bleeding is extremely rare after a simple screening colonoscopy. Patients using nonsteroidal anti-inflammatory medications, like aspirin and ibuprofen, and patients taking blood thinners, such as heparin and warfarin (coumadin), are at higher risk for bleeding complications. For this reason, aspirin and other nonsteroidal anti-inflammatory medications like ibuprofen (Advil™ or Motrin™) should ideally be stopped 2 weeks before colonoscopy. Coumadin should also be stopped several days before the procedure, but only under the strict guidance of a physician. You should absolutely not stop taking your coumadin unless you have been instructed to do so by your doctor. Nearly all cases of bleeding after polyp removal stop by themselves without further medical treatment, but severe cases may require blood transfusion. Rare cases of persistent bleeding may require additional interventions, like repeat colonoscopy, angiography, or even surgery.

Perforation through the bowel wall as a result of colonoscopy is even more rare, occurring in only 1 out of 1,000 procedures. It usually happens in one of two ways. The least traumatic is the small "microperforation" that results from excessive heat from the electric cautery used during polyp removal. This can generally be treated successfully with observation, diet restriction, and antibiotic therapy; surgery is usually not required. A more significant perforation can occur as the result of colonoscopic manipulation in a colon that has difficult bends, usually as a result of previous surgery. Although exceedingly rare, such tears require immediate surgical exploration and repair. In severe cases, a temporary stoma (loop of bowel brought out surgically through the abdominal wall) may be required.

22. What is virtual colonoscopy?

Virtual colonoscopy is a combination of computer and radiology technology. Like a barium enema, virtual colonoscopy is a radiologic screening test, but instead of using regular flat x-rays for images, it uses the computed tomographic (CT) scanner to generate computer images of the entire colon. After the colon is filled with air, a specialized CT scan of the colon is performed that generates multiple cross-sectional images of the abdomen. A computer program converts these x-ray images into a three-dimensional representation of the colon. As in a computer video game, your doctor can "walk" through this computer-generated image, looking for suspicious lesions.

The accuracy of virtual colonoscopy has been good in early simulations, especially for larger polyps. Studies have demonstrated that virtual colonoscopy can identify 90% of 1-cm polyps seen with colonoscopy, but only 25% of polyps smaller than 5 millimeters. Therefore, although it poses minimal risk for colonic injury, it is not yet ready to replace endoscopy. Other disadvantages are that it can be used only for diagnosis, and actual colonoscopy is required to evaluate all abnormal findings. And virtual colonoscopy still requires a full bowel preparation and the uncomfortable insufflation of gas into the colon. Virtual colonoscopy is also very expensive, especially when you realize that it doesn't allow the doctor to remove any polyps he or she might find. However, it is a useful tool for patients who cannot undergo colonoscopy and may have a future benefit for colorectal cancer screening.

23. Why isn't there a blood test that can identify patients with colon cancer?

It would be ideal if there were a simple blood test that could identify patients who are at risk for developing colorectal cancer or those who already have a cancer. Unfortunately, the search for a blood marker in colo-rectal cancer has not been as successful as it has been in other diseases.

The closest test available for colorectal surgery is the **carcinoembryonic antigen (CEA) level**. CEA is a protein created by the mucosa of normal gastrointestinal mucosal cells. An elevated CEA level is associated with colorectal cancer. However, although CEA is found predominantly in the colon and rectum, it appears in other organs as well. For this reason, elevations of CEA may not mean that colorectal cancer is present. For example, cancers of the breast, pancreas, stomach, bladder, thyroid, and lung can all cause elevated levels of CEA. Individuals with liver cirrhosis have elevated levels of CEA because of reduced metabolism in the diseased liver. CEA level is also elevated in long-term smokers. Studies performed during the 1970s showed that using the CEA as a screening test was inefficient. There were many false-positive results (when a test comes up positive, but it is really negative), leading to unnecessary invasive screening tests. CEA is therefore not used as a colorectal cancer screening test.

Carcinoembryonic antigen (CEA) level

A test to detect a protein that is often created by colon cancers.

CEA is predominantly used for follow-up after surgery for colorectal cancer. In some patients, a rising CEA level may be the first sign that the cancer has recurred. Once the level starts to rise, additional studies, including CT scanning, **positron emission tomographic (PET)** scanning (see Question 32), or colonoscopy can be performed to look for recurrent disease. CEA used as part of postoperative surveillance has been shown to detect recurrent disease approximately 5 months

Positron emission tomographic (PET)

Radiographic study that uses the abnormal sugar metabolism of cancer cells to identify metastatic deposits.

earlier than physical examination alone. The main role for the use of CEA testing is in long-term cancer follow-up.

24. OK. You have made your point that screening is vital for the prevention of colorectal cancer. As an average person, what kind of screening should I have?

Let's begin with the basics. As health care professionals, we realize that no one wants to go to the doctor for colorectal cancer screening. Digital rectal examination, rigid proctoscopy, and colonoscopy are uncomfortable procedures that some people find embarrassing. However, these tests are the key to the prevention, successful diagnosis, and treatment of colorectal cancer. The longer the delay in screening, the higher the chance that a small polyp, which initially may be easily removed, will grow larger and form a cancer.

Appropriate screening protocols for colorectal cancer have been in place since 1990 (Table 2). Recently, the American Cancer Society revised these guidelines by dividing patients into one of three groups: average, moderate, and high risk. We follow the recommendations of the American Society of Colon and Rectal Surgeons, which are similar to those of the American Cancer Society (Table 2).

Screening consists of a combination of fecal occult blood testing, flexible sigmoidoscopy, and colonoscopy. What kind of testing you will need depends on your risk of developing colorectal cancer. Average-risk patients are defined as people with no family history of colorectal cancer who do not have a personal history of colonic polyps and who have no concurrent medical syndromes like FAP, HNPCC, or inflammatory bowel disease (see Question 14). Moderate- to high-risk patients have a number of these additional risk factors. We discuss some of the more common recommendations below, and they are also summarized in Table 2.

Table 2 Screening guidelines of the American Society of Colon and Rectal Surgery

Risk	Procedure	Age at Onset (year)	Frequency
I. Low or average risk A. Asymptomatic—no risk factors B. Colorectal cancer in no first-degree relatives	Digital rectal exam AND one of the following:	50	Yearly
	Fecal occult blood testing and flexible sigmoidoscopy	50	FOBT yearly, flexible sigmoidoscopy every 5 years
	or Total colon exam (colonoscopy or double contrast enema and proctosigmoidoscopy)	50	Every 5–10 years
II. Moderate risk A. Colorectal cancer in first-degree relative, age 55 or younger, or two or more first-degree relatives of any ages	Colonoscopy	40, or 10 years before the youngest case in the family, whichever is earlier	Every 5 years
B. Colorectal cancer in a first-degree relative over the age of 55	Colonoscopy	50, or 10 years before the age of the youngest case, whichever is earlier	Every 5–10 years
C. Personal history of large polyps (>1 cm) or multiple colorectal polyps of any size	Colonoscopy	One year after polyp removal	If recurrent polyps, 1 year. If normal, 5 years
D. Personal history of colorectal malignancy—surveillance after resection for curative intent	Colonoscopy	One year after resection	If normal, 3 years. If still normal, 5 years. If abnormal, as above (continued)

(continued)

Table 2 continued

Risk	Procedure	Age at Onset (year)	Frequency
III. High risk			
A. Family history of hereditary adenomatous polyposis (FAP)	Flexible sigmoidoscopy; consider genetic counseling; consider genetic testing	12–14 (puberty)	Every 1–2 years
B. Family history of hereditary nonpolyposis cancer (HNPCC)	Colonoscopy; consider genetic counseling; consider genetic testing	21–40 40	Every 2 years Yearly
C. Inflammatory bowel disease			
1. Left-sided colitis	Colonoscopy	15th year of disease	Every 1–2 years
2. Pancolitis	Colonoscopy	8th year of disease	Every 1–2 years

Average Risk: Most of the population falls into the category of average risk. Screening for colorectal cancer should begin at age 50. One commonly recommended screening regime includes digital rectal examination and fecal occult blood testing annually, and flexible sigmoidoscopy every 5 years. Abnormal findings on FOBT or flexible sigmoidoscopy warrant examination of the entire colon by colonoscopy. An alternative method of screening for average-risk individuals is colonoscopy every 5 to 10 years. Although this method of screening has not been extensively studied, indirect evidence suggests that this technique is effective. Recent studies have suggested that colonoscopy is more effective because it can evaluate the right side of the colon, which is not visualized by sigmoidoscopy. This has been the stimulus for a change in government policy; Medicare now covers the use of colonoscopy for cancer screening. If you are found to have polyps on colonoscopy, you become elevated into a higher-risk group and will require additional screening in the future.

Personal History of Adenomatous Colorectal Polyps: Once you have adenomatous polyps in your colon, you are at higher risk for developing more polyps or even cancer. For this reason, you will need more screening. The National Polyp Study clearly demonstrated the efficacy of colonoscopy in preventing cancer in patients with a history of colonic polyps. They repeated colonoscopy in these patients and demonstrated that the incidence of cancer was 90% less than the incidence in a group that had not undergone such screening! Additionally, although colonoscopy is very accurate in identifying polyps, approximately 10% to 15% of small polyps may be missed during the initial colonoscopy. Therefore, patients who are found to have large adenomatous polyps or multiple polyps on colonoscopy should undergo a repeat examination in a year's time. If the repeat examination demonstrates a clear colon, screening can then be performed every 5 years.

Family History of Colorectal Cancer or Adenoma: People with a first-degree relative with colorectal cancer or colorectal adenomas should undergo more vigorous screening because of their increased risk of colorectal cancer. Screening should begin at age 40, or 10 years before the age of the earliest diagnosed cancer, whichever is earlier. The frequency of screening can follow the guidelines for average-risk patients, except that it should be started earlier. If you have a strong family history, with many first-degree relatives with colorectal cancer, some of whom may have developed them at a young age, you may have one of the hereditary non-polyposis syndromes (Lynch syndromes). You should seek out genetic counseling at an institution that specializes in such matters.

History of Inflammatory Bowel Disease: Individuals with inflammatory bowel disease need a screening colonoscopy that is started 8 years after the initial diagnosis. Repeat colonoscopies are necessary every 1 to 2 years thereafter. During these examinations, multiple random mucosal biopsy specimens need to be performed almost every 10 centimeters to look for occult (hidden) neoplasia. Proctocolectomy (surgical removal of the colon and rectum) is required in patients with low- or high-grade dysplasia because of their high incidence of occult colorectal cancer.

History of FAP: Patients and families with a family -history of FAP ideally need to be followed-up at in-stitutions that can recommend appropriate genetic counseling and workup. When genetic testing is not possible, flexible sigmoidoscopy should begin at age 12 and be repeated every 1 to 2 years until age 40. Once polyps are identified on sigmoidoscopy and the diagnosis of FAP is confirmed, then total proctocolectomy (surgical removal of the colon and rectum) should be discussed. Additionally, because people with FAP are at increased risk of duodenal polyps, upper endoscopy should be performed when FAP is initially diagnosed, and every 1 to 3 years thereafter.

History of HNPCC (Hereditary Nonpolyposis Colon Cancer): Patients suspected to have HNPCC should undergo screening beginning at age 21. Because of the incidence of right-sided cancers in this syndrome, flexible sigmoidoscopy is not adequate, and a full colonoscopy is necessary. A colonoscopy should be repeated every 2 years until age 40, and then yearly thereafter. Genetic screening can help identify patients with the genetic mutations that occur in people with HNPCC. Screening for associated tumors is also recommended.

Personal History of Colorectal Cancer: Patients who have had surgery for colorectal cancer should undergo a repeat colonoscopy 1 year later. After a normal study, routine surveillance every 3 years can begin. Patients who have had **low anterior resection** (see Question 36) for rectal cancer may undergo more frequent examination with either rigid proctoscopy or flexible sigmoidoscopy. Additional follow-up is discussed in later sections.

Low anterior resection
Resection of the lower rectum through a lower midline abdominal incision.

Screening is the key for early diagnosis of colorectal cancer, and it uses a combination of fecal occult blood testing, sigmoidoscopy, and colonoscopy. However, based on recent studies, initial examination and follow-up with colonoscopy has become the preferred method of screening among the average-risk population. So if you meet the average-risk criteria, are over 50 years old, and have not yet had your colonoscopy, don't delay!

25. Should I see a gastroenterologist or a colorectal surgeon for screening?

A **gastroenterologist** is a medical doctor specializing in disorders of the GI tract, most commonly peptic ulcer disease, hepatitis, and inflammatory bowel disease. Gastroenterologists perform endoscopy of the upper and lower GI tract.

Gastroenterologist
Medical doctor who specializes in disorders of the gastrointestinal tract.

Colorectal surgeons

Physicians who specialize in surgery for benign and malignant disorders of the colon and rectum; they also perform endoscopy of the lower GI tract.

Polypectomy

Surgical removal of polyps.

Colorectal surgeons specialize in surgery for benign and malignant disorders of the colon and rectum, and they also perform endoscopy of the lower GI tract. Colorectal surgeons treat benign problems of the anal canal, such as hemorrhoids and abscesses. In addition, they operate to remove both colon cancer and rectal cancer. Many colorectal surgeons are also skilled in laparoscopic techniques for colon surgery.

Surgeons and gastroenterologists both perform screening colonoscopy and colonoscopic **polypectomy** (surgical removal of polyps) and are both appropriate doctors for cancer screening. If surgery is required, your gastroenterologist will refer you to a surgeon.

26. I am worried that if I have a colonoscopy and my doctor finds a polyp, I will need surgery. Do all polyps need to be removed with major surgery?

Most polyps can be removed with techniques used during a colonoscopy.

Absolutely not! Most polyps can be removed with techniques used during a colonoscopy. Special instruments that biopsy, remove, or destroy polyps can be passed through small ports in the colonoscope. These use electrical currents to cauterize the tissue and minimize bleeding.

The primary risk of removing polyps colonoscopically is bleeding after the polyp is removed. People with bleeding disorders or those taking aspirin or other NSAIDs (nonsteroidal anti-inflammatory drugs) are at the highest risk for bleeding. If you are taking the blood thinner coumadin, you would need to consult your doctor about whether to stop taking it for several days before your colonoscopy to prevent bleeding from the surgical site. Another, rare (< 1%) risk is perforation of the colon wall. This can be a serious consequence and, depending on its severity, may require immediate surgery.

Most polyps can be removed via the colonoscope. However, some polyps that are located in difficult sections of the colon or are very large cannot be removed in this way. Because the right side of the colon is quite thin, large polyps here often cannot be removed because of the risk of colonic perforation. In these cases, an abdominal operation may be required to remove the colonic section containing the polyp. Laparoscopic techniques can also be used (see Question 42).

27. After having a colonoscopy, how long will it take before I know whether the polyp contained cancer or not?

After your colonoscopy, your doctor will briefly discuss the results with you or your chaperone. Because the effects of the anesthesia may linger for a short while, you may not remember much of what the doctor tells you. Be sure to call your physician during the next few days if you have any questions. Polyps removed during colonoscopy are sent for pathological evaluation (examination under a microscope), and final reports are usually available within several days. Most polyps are benign (not cancerous). Microscopic examination will determine the nature of the polyps and whether dysplasia (abnormal cell growth) or carcinoma (cancer) is present. Dysplastic polyps are treated with colonoscopic removal. Invasive cancers may require additional surgery (see Question 29).

PART FOUR

Treatment

What is a cancer's stage?

If my cancerous polyp was totally removed by colonoscopy, why might I still need to have surgery?

After being diagnosed with colorectal cancer, how long can I wait before having surgery?

More . . .

PREOPERATIVE WORKUP

28. What is a cancer's stage?

As doctors, there are several reasons it is important for us to have a standardized language for characterizing colorectal cancers. First of all, and most importantly, your prognosis depends on the extent and the spread of your cancer when it is first diagnosed. Tumors that have spread (metastasized) to other organs are both more aggressive and more advanced than small tumors that are limited to the bowel wall. Secondly, a consistent system allows us to pass on vital information to other doctors and to maintain an accurate treatment plan. It allows us to determine which patients should undergo investigation with surgical protocols and chemotherapy trials. For example, less advanced tumors are treated only with surgery, whereas less advanced tumors with high risk features and more advanced tumors may require a combination of surgery and chemotherapy. The most advanced tumors do not render themselves to surgery and thus only chemotherapy is appropriate for them. Tumor staging is the language doctors use to describe the nature of a tumor, as well as the extent of local and distant spread.

Tumor staging is based on three criteria: the tumor (T) depth, the evidence of lymph node (N) spread, and finally, the presence or absence of metastases (M). These three fundamentals form the TNM system for staging colorectal cancer (Tables 3 and 4).

Table 3 TNM staging chart

T		N		M	
0	Isolated to the mucosa	0	No evidence of lymph node spread	0	No evidence of lymph node spread
1	Into, but not through, the submucosa	1	Spread to 1–3 lymph nodes	1	Spread to 1–3 lymph nodes
2	Into but not through the muscle layer	2	Spread to greater than 3 lymph nodes	X	Spread to greater than 3 lymph nodes
3	Through the muscle layer into surrounding tissues	X	Unknown lymph node spread		Unknown lymph node spread
4	To adjacent organs				

Table 4 Overall tumor stage

	T	N	M
Stage I	1,2	0	0
Stage II	3,4	0	0
Stage III	Any	1,2	0
Stage IV	Any	Any	1

Abbreviations: T, tumor; N, node; M, metastasis.

T (Tumor Depth): The T stage identifies the extent that the tumor has invaded the bowel wall. The smaller the number, the less invasion there is. A T0 lesion is still a benign lesion, with abnormal changes identified only in the mucosa, whereas a T4 lesion has invaded the wall and into adjacent (nearby) organs.

N (Lymph Nodes): N describes the number of lymph nodes that contain cancerous spread. N0 means that no lymph nodes in the **pathology** specimen contained any cancer. Nx means that the number of positive lymph nodes is unknown. For example, if a cancer is staged during physical examination before surgery, it is impossible to determine the status of the lymph nodes. Until this is known, the stage is considered Nx.

Pathology
The branch of science that studies the nature of disease processes.

M (Metastases): M defines whether there is any metastatic spread to other organs.

The overall tumor stage is summarized in Table 4.

To read this table, look at the T, N, M headings at the top. Under each column are numbers or the word "any." The first entry under "T" reads 1, 2, and the entries under "N" and "M" are both zero. This means that if the tumor is confined to the bowel wall (T1 or T2) but no nodes have cancer and no metastases are present, the cancer is classified as Stage I. A cancer that extends beyond the bowel wall (T3 or T4), but when no cancer is present in the lymph nodes or anywhere else (metastases), is a Stage II. And so on.

Your doctor may refer to your cancer as a Dukes A, B, or C. This is an older staging system still used by many surgeons today. Dukes A, B, and C are synonymous with TNM Stages I, II, and III.

Staging is crucial in order to determine treatment options. Stage I colon cancers are usually treated with surgery alone, and Stage III cancers often are treated with both surgery and chemotherapy. Staging is therefore an important aspect of the preoperative workup. Many tests will be ordered to determine the correct stage before surgery. CT scans, chest x-rays, ultrasound, and PET scans (see Question 32) are all useful examinations to determine the extent of cancer spread. However, the actual staging will not be accurate until after surgery and pathological (microscopic) examination of the specimen.

In addition to the staging classifications described above certain features of the tumor help oncologists set apart a low risk from a high risk tumor. These features are described in the pathologist report and are taken into consideration when determining the most appropriate course of treatment. Less advanced tumor with any of the following high risk features is recommended to be viewed as a more advanced tumor. Some hish risk features are intervention with major veins, perforation of the bowel, and fewer than 12 lymph nodes after surgery.

It is important that you understand these concepts and keep in mind the criteria listed in the charts and the tumor features so that you can discuss treatment options and prognosis intelligently with your doctor. It may help to have a copy of the criteria with you for your appointment. We frequently refer to this staging system throughout the remainder of the book, so you may wish to mark this page and glance back at it from time to time.

29. If my cancerous polyp was totally removed by colonoscopy, why might I still need to have surgery?

There are prospects for cure in less advanced colorectal cancer cases when surgery removes the tumor in its entirety. Although adjuvant (nonsurgical) therapies like chemotherapy and radiation therapy can improve survival after surgery, they are not substitutes for surgical removal. Recent advances have shown some benefit in pre-treating the tumor with some chemotherapy prior to surgery to make the tumor smaller and thus easier to remove with surgery. Therefore, if any cancerous tissue is left behind after colonoscopic removal of a polyp, treatment is not adequate and surgery will be necessary.

For example, any polyp that cannot be removed completely by colonoscopy because of its size or location needs to be surgically removed. This seems obvious if the polyp contains cancer, but adenomatous (benign) polyps that can only be partially removed by colonoscopy also require surgery. Any part of the polyp left behind may contain malignant cells. The only way to tell without question whether a polyp contains cancer cells, and to confirm a benign diagnosis, is with total removal and microscopic examination. On the other hand, if a polyp is totally removed by colonoscopy and is found to contain only dysplasia or **carcinoma in situ** (precancerous change in the cells), then you do not require additional surgery. These abnormalities are confined to the mucosa of the bowel wall, and there is absolutely no chance for lymph node spread. Once they are removed, you are cured; however, you will need more frequent screening in the future to guard against new cancers forming.

Carcinoma in situ
Malignant cells that are confined to the colonic or rectal mucosa but do not invade the underlying submucosa.

Polyps that have been totally removed by colonoscopy but are found to contain a tiny focus of invasive cancer require further discussion. Even if this kind of polyp has been completely removed, you still may need surgery. This is a key point in understanding the management of colorectal cancer. Because the early cancer in the polyp has invaded the submucosa, there is a chance it may have spread into the nearby lymph nodes, and colonoscopic polyp surgery does not remove these nodes. They can be removed only by surgical removal of the part of the colon that contained the polyp along with its mesentery, where the lymph nodes reside. The recommendation for surgery in this situation is based on weighing the risk that lymph node metastasis will be present against the risk of surgery itself. In many cases, after the polyp is analyzed under the microscope, the risk of lymph node spread is judged to be so low that the risk of surgery may be greater than that of observation alone; in these cases, surgery may not be recommended. In other cases, however, the chance of lymph node metastasis can be higher because of microscopic features identified within the polyp once it has been removed and analyzed; in these cases, surgery is generally recommended. The risk of lymph node spread depends on the type of polyp present and its microscopic features, the adequacy of cancer removal, and the depth of cancer invasion into the submucosa. Your surgeon will review the microscopic slides with a pathologist and will make a recommendation based on these factors (Table 5). Aggressive tumors that have been inadequately removed colonoscopically will re-quire additional surgery.

Due to the variety of treatment approaches—surgery alone, or a combination of surgery and chemotherapy—it is important for the patient to seek the opinion of both the oncologist and the surgeon in advance of undertaking any particular treatment. Involving the oncologist prior to the surgery will ensure that if there is any benefit from pre-operative chemotherapy, he or she is able to recommend it on time.

Table 5 Factors determining recommendations for or against surgery after polyp removal

	Polyp contains dysplasia or "in-situ" cancer	Polyp contains invasive cancer
Polyp partially removed	Surgery	Surgery
Polyp completely removed	No Surgery	Depends on microscopic findings

30. After being diagnosed with colorectal cancer, how long can I wait before having surgery?

Although your surgery may take place relatively quickly, you should not feel concerned if your surgeon delays it for a few weeks. In general, colorectal cancers are slow-growing tumors, and the risk for spread during this time is low. Therefore, if your surgery is delayed a short time, this will not affect your chance for cure. During this time, any additional preoperative workup will be completed and medical and cardiology consultations may be scheduled. Patients with rectal cancer may be evaluated by a medical oncologist and radiation oncologist to determine whether chemo-therapy and radiation therapy could be beneficial before surgery. The need for either treatment depends on the stage of the rectal cancer. Preoperative treatments help to shrink the size of rectal cancers, allowing for more complete surgical resection, reducing the risk of local recurrence, and increasing the chance for **sphincter-saving surgery** (see Questions 44, 50, and 54).

You should not feel concerned if your surgeon delays it for a few weeks.

Sphincter-saving surgery

Surgery for removal of a rectal cancer that is able to spare the sphincter muscles and therefore avoid a permanent colostomy.

Occasionally, immediate surgery is needed for very large colorectal tumors. Advanced tumors like these can block the colon, causing the bowel to expand as it fills with waste that can't be pushed past the blockage. As the colon expands, the risk for perforation (splitting) of the bowel increases, and this can be a life-threatening emergency. Even tumors that only partially block the colon can be a problem because they limit the effectiveness of the preoperative bowel cleansing routine. For this reason, earlier surgery may reduce the need for a temporary stoma. Many people think that surgeons only "want to cut," and they may feel pressured if their doctor recommends urgent surgery. Please understand that nothing could be further from the truth. In general, surgeons have your best interest at heart, and in order to prevent serious complications, earlier surgery may be necessary.

31. How can I get my surgery done now? I have just started a new job, and my kids are going to college. How can I afford to take 6 months off from work?

Being diagnosed with colorectal cancer can be a daunting experience. You go to your doctor complaining of rectal bleeding, thinking it is just your hemorrhoids acting up, and you leave with the diagnosis of a life-threatening illness that requires surgery, possibly an **ostomy** (a surgically created opening from the inside to the outside of the body), 5 weeks of radiation, and 6 months of chemotherapy! How can anyone be expected to cope with this well? Cancer doesn't fit into your schedule, especially at a time when your finances may already be strapped.

Ostomy
A surgically created opening from the inside to the outside of the body.

But try not to get overwhelmed during this initial office visit. Everything seems worse when you are sitting across the table from your physician and the words stoma, chemotherapy, and surgery are all mentioned in the same sentence. Although procrastination is not prudent, a short delay will in no way affect your ability to beat this disease. You can take time to organize your life and finances, and build a network of social support. Although you will be out of working condition for about 4 to 6 weeks after surgery, many people tolerate adjuvant (nonsurgical, supplemental) treatments like chemotherapy and radiation therapy very well and continue to work part time or even full time, depending on the nature of their jobs. Many support systems are already in place to help you with your battle. Don't give up. In the last section of this book, we discuss ways to improve communication with the medical team, and methods of reducing your distress, including addressing work concerns, financial matters, and family issues. Step by step, you can learn how to better cope with this disease.

Take time to organize your life and finances, and build a network of social support.

Kate's Comment:

I didn't have much choice in either of my surgeries. Both tumors were large and partially blocking the colon. Hidden bleeding had left me very anemic. I was hospitalized immediately while x-rays, colonoscopy, and other tests were done, and the surgery was performed within days. However, I couldn't imagine letting the tumor grow because surgery was inconvenient. The risk of spread to my liver or lungs was just too great. The sooner the cancer is found and treated, the better. Besides, waiting for months would just prolong anxiety.

32. What additional tests will I need before surgery?

When you and your surgeon have decided on surgery, an additional series of tests or "workup" will begin. The goals of these tests are twofold. First, a combination of studies stage the tumor and determine the extent of its spread. The cancer stage at the time of diagnosis determines treatment. Clearly, the treatment of a colon cancer that has spread to the liver will differ significantly from the treatment of a small tumor that is limited to the bowel wall.

A chest x-ray study will be performed to evaluate the lungs for cancer spread. This routine examination is very sensitive in identifying lung nodules. It can also reveal evidence of lung or heart disease and is therefore a standard preoperative examination before any major surgery. CT scans of the abdomen and pelvis will be performed to assess the liver and peritoneal (abdominal) cavity for evidence of cancer spread (see Question 33). Sometimes a CT scan of the chest is included with the CT of the abdomen, and a simple chest x-ray study may then be unnecessary. PET scanning uses a radioactive form of glucose (sugar) to identify tumor deposits. Although it is very sensitive in identifying occult (hidden) metastases that are not seen on x-ray or CT studies, PET scanning is not yet the standard of care for preoperative cancer staging.

Additional tests are performed to evaluate your overall state of health and to assess your risk for surgery.

Besides the preoperative staging of the cancer, additional tests are performed to evaluate your overall state of health and to assess your risk for surgery. Surgery is a stress on the body and can exacerbate underlying lung, heart, or kidney problems, so screening tests can be helpful in identifying patients who are at risk for difficulty during and after surgery. These teststest-stests can be performed at the hospital or with your private physician, and are referred to as preadmission tests. A panel of blood tests will be collected, including a complete blood count (CBC), blood chemistry, and coagulation profile. A complete blood count measures circulating blood counts, including the red blood cell, the white blood cell, and the platelet counts. All these cells are crucial in day-to-day activity. Red cells carry oxygen in the body and are vital for tissue oxygenation. Colon cancers tend to cause microscopic bleeding, and therefore, the red blood count is commonly low in these patients. In severe cases, blood transfusion may be necessary after surgery or even before. Because **platelets** are responsible for normal blood clotting, the platelet count is a necessary preoperative test. Without a history of abnormal bleeding in the past, including excessive nosebleeds or bleeding gums, it is unlikely that platelet counts will be abnormal. Nevertheless, this must be checked beforehand to reduce the risk of bleeding during surgery. Serum chemistries calculate blood electrolytes, such as sodium and potassium; the levels of these electrolytes can be unusually high or low in patients taking blood pressure and other types of medications and would need to be corrected before surgery. The coagulation profile measures the efficiency of blood clotting factors because blood clotting can be abnormal in patients with hemophilia or other factor deficiencies. Finally, women of childbearing age require a preoperative pregnancy test to make sure that they are not pregnant.

Platelets

Blood cells responsible for blood clotting.

An EKG (electrocardiogram) is a screening test that evaluates the heart. It can reveal signs of atherosclerotic heart disease (narrowing or hardening of the arteries), which is a significant risk for major surgery. EKG findings consistent with previous heart attacks or current cardiac ischemia (insufficient blood flow that results in inadequate tissue oxygenation) are evidence of atherosclerotic disease of the coronary arteries. An abnormal EKG warrants additional workup that is coordinated by your primary physician and possibly a cardiologist. Once the workup is completed, and additional therapy initiated if needed, you will be "cleared" for surgery.

Pati's Comment:

The usual tests ordered before surgery are a chest x-ray, CT scan, EKG, and blood work—kidney, liver, glucose, red and white blood counts, and a CEA. It can be helpful to get a baseline CEA prior to surgery to compare with future CEA levels. It was a flurry of tests; I was so busy, I think I was operating on autopilot at the time.

33. What is a CT scan? Is this the same as an MRI scan?

Treatment for colorectal cancer is based on accurate preoperative staging. CT scanning (**computed tomography**, also known as "CAT scanning") is the current standard preoperative evaluation of the liver for evidence of cancer spread. CT scanning uses x-rays to create digital images of the abdominal organs. These images can show local tumor growth and detect spread of the cancer (metastases) in the abdomen or liver. CT is a very sensitive test that identifies over 80% of liver metastases. In order to enhance the quality of the images, special contrast agents are given by mouth and also intravenously (into the veins). For preoperative evaluation, intravenous contrast is necessary to identify liver metastases.

Computed tomography (CT)
Radiologic examination that utilizes x-rays to generate a two-dimensional computer image of the area scanned.

CT is a routine test, and thousands are performed daily in the United States. However, allergic reactions to the intravenous contrast can occur in some people; these reactions range from a simple skin rash to severe respiratory and cardiac distress. The risk of allergic complications is exceedingly low, occurring in 0.2% to 0.4% of patients, and these complicagtions occur more frequently in patients with food allergies to shellfish. Most of these reactions are minor, and they are easily treated with simple medications, like antihistamines. However, intravenous contrast agents can also cause temporary kidney dysfunction. Although such complications can be severe, the kidney function generally returns to normal with time and conservative treatment. Kidney complications occur more frequently in patients with preexisting kidney disease. Be sure to raise any concerns you have with your radiologist before your examination.

Magnetic resonance imaging (MRI)

A diagnostic radiology study that uses nuclear technology.

Magnetic resonance imaging (MRI) is also used to image the organs of the abdomen and pelvis. MRI is performed inside a tunnel-shaped machine, and the patient is positioned so that the organ to be imaged is inside the tunnel. MRI takes longer to perform than CT scanning, and the tunnel can be unsettling for some patients, particularly people who experience claustrophobia. Because MRI uses strong magnets to obtain images, all metal objects need to be removed from the room. If you have had surgery before and metal implants were placed (artificial hips or joints), you may not be able to undergo an MRI.

MRI does not require iodinated contrast material (the kind used for CT scans) and can therefore be used in patients who are allergic to the contrast material. Unfortunately, although imaging of the liver is excellent, MRI imaging of the remainder of the abdomen is not as good as that provided by CT scanning. MRI is also more expensive. For these reasons, MRI is not a routine part of the preoperative workup of colorectal cancer. It is used as an additional test to clarify the nature of unclear lesions seen on CT scan and to further evaluate advanced rectal cancers and recurrent disease. It is not a substitute for CT scanning.

34. What kind of preparation will I need for surgery? Will I need to come into the hospital? How should I pack for my hospital stay?

Colorectal surgery, like colonoscopy, requires a complete bowel preparation the day before. This is necessary to prevent postoperative complications and should not be taken lightly. A bowel preparation, such as GoLYTELY™ or Fleet® Phospho-soda®, combined with oral antibiotics, is the standard regimen used to minimize the amount of bacteria in the colon. Common antibiotic choices include neomycin and metronidazole (Flagyl™) or neomycin and erythromycin. You will be given detailed instructions by your surgeon on when you should take these medications before surgery. Like the preparation before colonoscopy, you should continue to take the bowel preparation until your bowel movements are a transparent liquid; this signifies that the cleansing has been adequate. Patients with large tumors may require bowel preparation that is spread slowly over 2 or 3 days. During this time, your diet will be limited to liquids only. Make an extra effort to keep up with your fluid intake during the bowel preparation, because it is very easy to become dehydrated.

Make an extra effort to keep up with your fluid intake during the bowel preparation, because it is very easy to become dehydrated.

Adequate bowel preparation is necessary because it reduces the risk of postoperative infection. As you can imagine, the colon normally contains extremely high concentrations of bacteria. Spread of these bacteria outside the colon can lead to postoperative infection. The most common area for infection is the skin, with the risk of wound complications approaching 5% to 10%. However, bowel cleansing routines have significantly lowered the risk of wound infections after surgery. When cleansing is incomplete, the risk of problems with the bowel **anastomosis** (the surgical connection between 2 loops of intestine) increases, and infection can occur within the abdomen. If you are having trouble with your bowel preparation, call your surgeon the day before surgery rather than risk problems the morning of surgery. If you cannot tolerate the taste, are becoming nauseated, or feel that the preparation is simply not working, do not wait until the morning of surgery to tell your doctor. Other bowel preparation techniques are available that may be more easily tolerated.

Anastomosis
Surgical connection between ends of bowel.

Patients are usually no longer admitted to the hospital the day before surgery for preparation and workup. Therefore, you will need to complete your bowel preparation at home and come to the hospital the morning of surgery. Today's hospitals are geared toward same-day surgery and will give you specific instructions regarding the time you will need to arrive in the morning.

During the bowel preparation before surgery, your diet will be limited to clear liquids only. In addition, you cannot eat any food or drink any time after midnight before surgery. If you come to the hospital the morning of surgery with a full stomach, you will be at considerable risk for aspiration (choking on regurgitated food) during anesthesia. Do not have anything to eat or drink the morning of your surgery, not even your morning bowel of cereal, a slice of toast, or your cup of coffee! Doing so will only delay your surgery because your anesthesiologist and surgeon will absolutely not allow you to undergo elective surgery if you have eaten. Eating or drinking will delay your surgery a minimum of 6 hours; otherwise, surgery would pose an unnecessary risk to you. However, you should take your usual morning medications, if so directed by your doctor, with small sips of water (see Question 35).

Be practical, and use your common sense.

You will want to be prepared for a brief stay in the hospital when you arrive. Be practical, and use your common sense. Don't bring expensive valuables, fancy clothing, or lots of cash with you. But you should bring a small case of supplies. You will be bedridden only for the day of your surgery; after that, you will be quickly encouraged to move and walk around. Hospital gowns are far from flattering and can be quite revealing, so a pair of loose-fitting pajamas or a nightgown, as well as slippers with no-slip soles, will be useful. Remember that there still may be a small amount of leakage from the incision after surgery, and even with a sterile dressing this can stain clothes. Don't bring your cherished clothing that may get damaged.

Toiletries like a toothbrush, hairbrush, deodorant, perfumes, and colognes may help you to feel more "human" after surgery.

However, contact lenses are not permitted during surgery, so wear your glasses and save your lenses for the postoperative period. Leave your wallet and other valuables with your family before surgery, but keep a small amount of money or a single credit card with you for the telephone and movie rentals. You may also want to bring a good book, some magazines, or small craft projects to keep you busy during the latter part of you hospital admission, when you start to feel better. Refer to Part 5 of this book to learn about coping with the stress of surgery and hospitalization.

Pati's Comment:

You are going to be spending a lot of time resting, so you don't need to bring much with you. Pack for comfort, bring a robe, slippers, a few toiletries such as lip balm, lotion, talcum powder, toothbrush and toothpaste, travel-size shampoo, a notepad and pen, and a magazine. In hindsight, I wish I had brought along a couple of pins or clips for the back of the hospital gown! I was advised not to bring my own sleepwear, in case it got stained.

Kate's Comment:

Hospital gowns, while sometimes skimpy and faded, are easy to keep changed and clean and have special fasteners to accommodate IV tubing. So I leave my nighties home, but bring a pretty robe and slippers because walking is so important to recovery.

I always bring along a Walkman-style tape player with extra batteries. Listening to music or a book on tape eases my worries and passes my slow hospital time. Books on tape are relaxing in the first couple of days when reading isn't easy because of pain medication and the fatigue of a major operation.

Although the hospital supplies soap and toothpaste, I bring my own so I can have the extra luxury of rose or lavender in the stinky hospital room, and I pack my own special brand of body wash and shampoo for the wonderful day when enough tubes and stitches come out so I can have a shower. Doing what I could for myself in the hospital was very important, even if it was as small as washing my face with sweet soap. It gave me a sense of control in a place without much personal control and encouraged me to begin moving forward.

35. What if I have other medical problems, like diabetes, high blood pressure, or angina? Can I still have surgery? Should I continue to take my medications the day of surgery?

A patient with other medical conditions, particularly conditions that are potentially life- threatening, faces an increased risk from surgery. However, because most colorectal cancer patients are generally older, these fairly common problems are routinely managed by your surgical team. Advanced age alone is not a risk factor for abdominal surgery. Patients in their 70s and 80s routinely undergo colon surgery without complication. Do not compromise your care because you think, "I am too old to have major surgery." Age is an issue only when it is associated with other health problems that increase risk. The key to preventing complications is to identify these risks beforehand so that appropriate measures can be taken. However, not all medical problems are clearly apparent and, like cancer, can be occult (hidden). This is the reason for your workup before surgery, and the direction the workup takes will be dictated by your surgeon and primary care physician.

The key to preventing complications is to identify these risks beforehand.

Hypertension

High blood pressure.

Angina

Chest pain that results from atherosclerotic heart disease.

Myocardial infarction

Damage to heart cells as a result of decreased blood flow; a heart attack.

Cardiac (Heart) Problems: Because general anesthesia and abdominal surgery place physical stresses on the body, the risk during surgery is most serious for those with heart problems. Patients with a history of heart disease, including severe **hypertension** (high blood pressure), **angina** (chest pain), or **myocardial infarction** (heart attack), need additional workup before surgery. Patients without a complicated medical history and a normal EKG rarely need additional studies. Based on your clinical symptoms, your surgeon may have you consult a cardiologist for evaluation preoperatively. Intensive cardiac workup begins with a stress test, which screens for cardiac **ischemia** (loss of blood flow).

Ischemia
Insufficient blood flow resulting in inadequate tissue oxygenation.

An exercise stress test involves walking on a treadmill while special monitors to record heart function. Patients who cannot perform a physical stress test because of problems like arthritis or asthma need to undergo a chemical (pharmacologic) stress test instead. During a pharmacologic stress test, intravenous stimulants are given that speed up the heart while ultrasound or nuclear scans evaluate cardiac function and blood flow. If the results of these noninvasive screening tests are abnormal, additional workup with more invasive and therapeutic examinations, like an angiogram, might be needed. With current techniques for screening and intervention, however, the risk of heart problems during and after surgery has fallen significantly.

Pulmonary (Lung) Problems: Lung complications during surgery, although often less severe than cardiac complications, occur more frequently in patients with underlying lung disease like emphysema. The most important step in preventing lung problems is to stop smoking! If you stop smoking just a few weeks before surgery, you will significantly reduce your risk for complications like pneumonia. Breathing problems occur because the pain from an abdominal incision limits your ability to take deep breaths after surgery ("splinting"); this can be a significant problem in patients with underlying lung disease. A pulmonologist (a doctor specializing in diseases of the lung) may be consulted to help in the postoperative period. Pulmonary function tests that measure the absorptive capacity and functional reserve of the lungs will be performed.

If you stop smoking just a few weeks before surgery, you will significantly reduce your risk for complications like pneumonia.

You may be given a combination of oral and inhaled medications that optimize respiratory function before and after surgery. Additionally, you may be a candidate for **epidural anesthesia** (see Question 37), which can be more effective in limiting pain during the postoperative period. With less

Epidural anesthesia
Anesthesia that is administered via a small catheter that is inserted into the epidural space around the spinal cord.

pain, you can have less "splinting" and improved lung function. Finally, because a respirator is used during surgery, patients with severe emphysema may need longer ventilator support after surgery, as well as a brief stay in the intensive care unit. Discuss these issues with your surgeon before surgery.

Diabetes: Diabetes, like age, is not an independent risk factor for surgical complications. However, patients with long-standing diabetes are at increased risk for occult (hidden) cardiac and renal disease. If you have long-standing diabetes, additional preoperative testing and cardiac workup may be warranted.

Renal (Kidney) Problems: Patients with chronic renal failure who require hemodialysis present complicated problems during the perioperative period. Renal failure affects the body's ability to regulate fluids and electrolytes normally. During surgery, there are many fluid shifts due to blood loss and fluid replacement. In addition, patients with renal failure have abnormal platelets and abnormal blood clotting. Despite all these problems, surgery can be performed safely in patients with chronic renal failure. Your surgical team and nephrologist will carefully coordinate preoperative and postoperative management. You may be admitted to the hospital the day before for observation during your preoperative bowel preparation. In general, dialysis will be scheduled the day before surgery, and postoperative dialysis will be scheduled based on clinical examinations.

Although these disorders affect management during surgery, they do not mean you should not have surgery; they simply require a coordinated effort between you, your surgeon, and your medical internist. Careful workup is the key to preventing surgical complications.

It will also be important to continue taking your medications until the day of surgery. Although you will be limited to a liquid diet the day before, and although you will be fasting completely after midnight, in general you should continue to take your medications. However, there are exceptions to this rule. Make a point of asking your doctor which medications to take, which to avoid, and how long prior to surgery you should stop taking certain medications. Ask your doctor to provide you with written instructions, especially if you are taking more than one medication; do not rely on memory alone during this stressful time.

Ask your doctor to provide you with written instructions, especially if you are taking more than one medication; do not rely on memory alone during this stressful time.

Antihypertensive
Medication used to lower blood pressure.

Some examples of medications you should discuss with your doctor are:

Medications you SHOULD take: You should continue to take all **antihypertensives** (blood pressure medications), including beta blockers, angiotensin-converting enzyme (ACE) inhibitors, and diuretics (water pills), the morning of surgery with a sip of water. Antihypertensives help stabilize your blood pressure during surgery. Beta blockers decrease the risk of perioperative cardiac events in patients with atherosclerotic heart disease. Diuretics (water pills) help reduce your risk of congestive heart failure from fluid overload. However, diuretics can cause you to become too dehydrated when they are used in conjunction with the preoperative bowel preparation. For this reason, although in general you should take your medications the morning of surgery, if you do take diuretics, make sure to discuss this point with your surgeon.

Medications you SHOULD NOT take: You should stop taking NSAIDs (nonsteroidal anti-inflammatory drugs), which include aspirin, ibuprofen (Advil™, Motrin™, and others), and naproxen (Naprosyn™). These medications impair platelet function and can cause abnormal blood clotting. (Aspirin prevents heart attacks by preventing blood clots in the coronary arteries.) The effects of NSAIDs and aspirin last for about 2 weeks and should therefore be stopped 2 weeks before surgery.

Herbal preparations: Although you can buy these supplements over the counter without a prescription, many of these medications contain potent drugs that have effects on the whole body. For example, Ginkgo biloba affects blood clotting. You should discuss all your vitamin and herbal supplements with your physician. In general, however, you should stop taking them before surgery to prevent unknown drug interactions. Be aware that even some non-medical herbal preparations, such as teas, could have unwanted effects. So check out their potential effects before you take them.

Anticoagulant
Medication that inhibits normal blood clotting.

Coumadin: Coumadin is an **anticoagulant** that affects normal bleeding by reducing the amount of clotting factors produced by the liver. Coumadin's effect on the liver lasts about 4 or 5 days and needs to be stopped several days before surgery to prevent bleeding complications. During this time, you may need to switch to another anticoagulant, like heparin. Unlike coumadin, heparin's effects last only a few hours and can be "turned off" right before surgery. Heparin is either given intravenously, which requires hospitalization, or subcutaneously, on an outpatient basis. A hematologist (a doctor specializing in blood disorders) may be consulted to manage your perioperative anticoagulation. To prevent life-threatening complications, absolutely never stop taking your coumadin without specific instructions from your doctor.

Insulin
Hormone responsible for stabilizing blood sugar.

Antiglycemics (diabetic medications): If you have diabetes, you should continue taking your regular medications the day before surgery. However, you will not be eating the day of surgery, so oral antiglycemics and **insulin** should not be taken the morning of surgery to prevent your blood sugar from falling too low. Severe diabetics may need to take a smaller dose the morning of surgery, but this should be coordinated with your doctor.

Please remember that these are only general suggestions and cannot cover every possibility. You should discuss all of your medications with your doctors before surgery.

SURGERY

36. What kind of operation will I need for my colon cancer? How are these operations performed?

The location of the tumor within the colon will determine the kind of surgery you will have. Cancers of the rectum present additional technical and functional challenges and are discussed at length in later questions.

The goal of surgery is to remove the segment of colon that contains the tumor as well as the lymph nodes into which the area drains. Because cancer cells spread via the lymph channels to the lymph nodes, the lymph nodes also need to be removed to reduce the risk of colon cancer recurrence. Secondly, by evaluating the lymph nodes that are removed, we can accurately "stage" the tumor (see Question 28). Tumor staging is necessary to determine the need for additional treatment, like chemotherapy. Colon lymph nodes lie in the fatty tissue (mesentery) surrounding the blood vessels that supply the colon. The spread of cancer therefore has a fixed pattern that follows the blood supply to a segment of colon. Therefore, during surgery, the mesentery is removed all the way down to the beginning of the blood vessel that supplies blood to it. By removing this part of the mesentery, the surgeon is very likely to have removed a number of lymph nodes along with it. An adequate staging requires a minimum of 12 lymph nodes to be removed and evaluated, and the first pre-requisite for that is the adequate removal of mesentery.

Surgical removal (resection) of the colon is called a colectomy. Tumors on the right side of the colon require a right hemicolectomy, and tumors on the left side, a left hemicolectomy. Tumors in the sigmoid require a sigmoid colectomy. On average, about 12 to 18 inches of colon are removed in a normal resection, although this length varies depending on the patient's size and weight.

Colonic operations are usually performed through an incision that stretches above and below the belly button in the middle of your abdomen. Using **electrocautery**, a device that utilizes electricity to cut tissue, the colon is separated from its attachments to other organs and the abdominal wall. The mesentery and lymph nodes are removed. The colon section containing the cancer is removed, and the ends of the bowel are reconnected with an anastomosis (bowel connection). Anastomoses can be performed with hand-sewn stitches, however, most are now completed with special stapling devices. The abdominal cavity is then closed. The muscles of the abdominal wall are "rebuilt" using absorbable suture material that lasts several months, and the skin is closed with metallic staples. These staples are removed 7 to 10 days after surgery.

Electrocautery

Using electricity to destroy tissue.

37. What should I expect when I come into the operating room? What kind of anesthesia will I get?

On the day of surgery, you will arrive at the hospital preadmission area a couple of hours before your surgery is scheduled to start. All necessary paperwork will be completed, and you will then be taken to a preoperative holding area where you will get undressed and change into a hospital gown. During this time, you will be questioned by a variety of hospital staff regarding your past medical history, drug allergies, and the upcoming surgical procedure. Try not to get frustrated from the repetition; these questions are repeated to prevent mistakes.

Answer all of the anesthesiologist's questions thoroughly and honestly to prevent complications.

Your anesthesiologist or one of his or her associates will evaluate you in the holding area, and will explain to you the type of anesthesia you will be receiving during your surgery. Answer all of the anesthesiologist's questions thoroughly and honestly to prevent complications, and be sure to ask any questions that you have regarding your anesthesia. Then, you will sign an informed consent form stating that you understand the risks of anesthesia. Your surgeon will also see you in the holding area. Feel free to ask any last-minute questions you may have to put your mind at ease. You will need to sign a separate consent form for your surgery. Make sure that you are signing for the correct procedure!

You will then be taken into the operating room. To ensure sterility, everyone there will be wearing a head covering and a face mask. You will transfer onto the operating room table. There will be many people in the room, including the anesthesiologist, the surgeon, a circulating nurse, and a scrub nurse. X-ray images may be up on the viewing box in the room. Your anesthesiologist will place an intravenous (IV) line into your arm. This requires just a small skin prick. Special stockings will be placed on your legs that help prevent blood clots in your veins during surgery. EKG leads will be placed on your chest, and a blood pressure cuff will be wrapped around your arm. When all the monitoring is complete, anesthesia will be given through the IV line and you will fall asleep and won't remember anything until you wake later in the recovery room. During surgery, a Foley catheter (hollow tube used to drain urine) is placed in your bladder, and sometimes a **nasogastric tube** (a suction tube that extends through the nose down into the esophagus and stomach to drain stomach contents) is placed.

Nasogastric tube

Suction tube placed through the nose down into the esophagus and stomach to drain gastric contents.

Colon surgery requires general anesthesia. You will be completely asleep with a breathing tube placed in your windpipe and a ventilator controlling your breathing. General anesthesia provides muscle relaxation, pain control, and amnesia. You will have no memory of your surgery.

For some patients, the anesthesiologist may recommend epidural anesthesia for additional pain control. Epidural anesthesia uses a small **catheter** that is inserted into the space around the spinal cord. Anesthetics may then be administered directly to the sensory nerves arising from the spinal cord. For this reason, epidural anesthesia provides the best pain control, and less general anesthesia is needed during surgery. If fewer inhaled gases are used, general anesthesia is safer and bet-

Catheter

A hollow tube used to drain or inject fluid.

ter tolerated by patients. After surgery, the epidural catheter can be left in place and you can administer pain medication yourself using a special patient control device. Fewer oral pain medications are needed, so there is less nausea following surgery. The epidural anesthesia is often used to control pain during childbirth. It is a common procedure, very safe, and complications are rare. Any questions regarding epidural anesthesia can be discussed with your anesthesiologist before surgery.

After your surgery is complete, you will continue to be monitored in the recovery room for another hour or two. You should not be alarmed by the number of tubes and wires attached to you because these are normal postoperative monitors. When you are fully awake in the recovery room, your family will be able to see you briefly. Usually, people are transferred to the regular hospital floor later that day.

38. What are the risks of surgery?

The risks posed by colon cancer surgery are similar to the risks from any abdominal surgery. These include the risk from general anesthesia, bleeding that requires a blood transfusion, postoperative infection, and even death. Because of constant improvements in anesthesia and surgery, the risk of these complications continues to fall. However, surgical risk cannot always be exactly determined because a great deal depends on individual factors, such as initial patient health and the extent of local and distant tumor spread.

Having to undergo surgery can be a significant life experience. It is common to feel stressed or anxious about surgery. However, try to remember that surgery is always a trade-off between risk and benefit; a small risk must be taken to overcome the greater challenge of defeating cancer. We provide a list of possible complications of surgery so that you are aware of some of the potential risks and benefits. The risks may seem frightening and overwhelming. Remember, though, that the surgical benefits far outweigh the small number of rare complications.

Transfusion: During surgery, there is always a risk of hemorrhage (blood loss) that might require transfusion and carries the accompanying risk of viral transmission. Hepatitis B, hepatitis C, and the human immuno-deficiency virus (HIV) are the viral infections with the highest chance of causing disease. With current screening protocols, however, the risk of contracting a disease during blood transfusion today is extremely rare. The chance of receiving an infected unit of blood varies from one in 250,000 for hepatitis B to one in one million for HIV. Although the risk of receiving contaminated blood is so low, many individuals still want to donate autologous (their own) blood before surgery. Donating your own blood can be more complicated than you may think. Colorectal cancer patients tend to be anemic (have low blood counts), and therefore they may not be able to donate any blood, but may even need a transfusion before surgery. Family members can donate blood if they are the same blood type as you, but their donations will still need to undergo routine blood screening, which takes a few days. In general, with the small amount of blood that is lost during routine colorectal surgery, preoperative donations are rarely necessary.

Infection: The risk of infection increases after bowel surgery because the colon contains high concentrations of bacteria. As described previously, the use of preoperative bowel preparations significantly reduces the risk of postoperative infection. However, even with adequate cleansing, the risk of infection exists, most commonly in the skin, such as a wound infection. The incidence of wound infections approaches 5% to 10% in colon resections. Uncomplicated wound infections are easily treated by removing some of the skin staples and allowing for adequate drainage. Saline dressing changes performed three times a day promote wound healing from the inside out.

Infection inside the abdomen after surgery is much less common, but it can be a more serious complication requiring percutaneous (through the skin) drainage, a second operation, or possibly the placement of a temporary stoma. Every effort is made during surgery to reduce postoperative infection, using sterile techniques and special wound protectors.

Anastomotic Leak: When the bowel is connected together with an anastomosis, there is always risk that the edges can separate and leak intestinal contents. "Anastomotic leaks" occur in about 2% to 4% of colon surgeries, which is about half the risk of rectal surgery. Many leaks are small and noticeable only from radiologic exams. They do not cause significant body symptoms and can often be treated with observation (monitoring), dietary restriction, and intravenous antibiotics. Large leaks, however, can be life-threatening and require immediate surgical re-exploration and ostomy placement (see Question 46). Because of the risk of anastomotic leak in rectal anastomoses, many surgeons perform a temporary diverting ileostomy (stoma created with small bowel). Temporary ileostomies do not prevent leaking from the rectal anastomosis, however, they do protect against the infectious complications that this leak can cause.

Small Bowel Obstruction: During the healing process after abdominal surgery, scar tissue can form inside the abdominal cavity between loops of bowel. These attachments are called adhesions and are under constant change during the healing process. If a loop of small bowel twists around an adhesion, a bowel obstruction can result. Intestinal contents become blocked, causing abdominal bloating, nausea, and vomiting. Partial small bowel obstructions can be treated non-surgically, with IV fluids and a nasogastric tube used to suction out stomach contents to help relieve the blockage. A small number require abdominal surgery to remove the offending adhesion.

39. How long will I need to be in the hospital after routine colon surgery? What can I expect during my hospitalization?

After surgery, you will be hospitalized for about 5 to 7 days. The main reason for this is that after any kind of abdominal surgery, the intestines become "paralyzed" and do not work normally for about 5 to 7 days. This is called an intestinal ileus. During this time, you may feel slightly nauseous and can have a poor appetite. You may not eat or drink much, so IV fluids will be administered constantly so that you do not get dehydrated. The Foley catheter, which was placed during surgery, will remain inside your bladder so that accurate measurement of your urine output can be obtained and indirectly judge your overall fluid status. A nasogastric tube (running from your nostril to your stomach) may be placed during surgery to suction out stomach contents, thereby preventing nausea from a gastric ileus.

On the first day after surgery, you will be encouraged to get out of bed and walk around. This may be difficult because of the normal pain you will experience from the abdominal incision. You will receive pain medication intravenously (given through your vein), intramuscularly (injected into your muscle), or orally (taken by mouth). Another device, called **patient-controlled analgesia (PCA)**, allows you to self-administer intravenous doses of specific pain medications and is commonly used after colorectal surgery. The most significant downside of these narcotic medications is that they can prolong the ileus (bowel inactivity) after surgery, which is a good reason to use less pain medication. However, many patients are afraid to take too much medication because they think that they will get addicted, or even worse, overdose. These fears are unfounded. It is far more important for you to get out of bed and walk as much as possible as early as possible. PCA devices are accurately calibrated, and they limit the amount of pain medication you can receive. Even if you press the button every few minutes, the PCA device will administer only

Patient-controlled analgesia (PCA)

Pump connected to an intravenous line that allows pain medication to be self-administered by a patient.

Ileus

Delayed bowel function after abdominal surgery.

the appropriate amount of medication. You cannot overdose. Secondly, because the machine helps you administer these medications appropriately, you will not become addicted.

You will usually be started on a liquid diet 1 or 2 days after surgery. Every day, your doctor will evaluate your progress and will gradually allow you to eat soft foods and then normal food, depending on how well you tolerate the changes. Once you can pass gas and move your bowels, you are ready to return home.

Pati's Comment:

I asked the anesthesiologist to put the NG [nasogastric] tube and bladder catheter in after the anesthesia was given so I wouldn't feel it. I knew the NG tube would help prevent nausea after surgery, but I sure wasn't looking forward to being awake while it was put in place. This was the first surgery with an NG tube and the first time that I didn't experience nausea afterward.

I knew the more I walked and moved around, the quicker the colon would start functioning. Who knew that passing gas could be such a cause of celebration? But it meant that I could start enjoying a liquid diet again. I walked my way right out of the hospital, and I went home 4 days after surgery.

40. Will I damage the incision if I get out of bed after surgery? Will I have a large scar?

You should not worry about hurting yourself with early activity after surgery. Although it will be uncomfortable to move around immediately, you will be encouraged on the first postoperative day to get out of bed and walk. If you feel too weak, it is important to make an effort to even just sit in a chair. The most important job you have as a patient is to get up and around the day after surgery; early activity will reduce your risk of pneumonia or a clot in your legs, and it also causes your bowel function to return more quickly to

The most important job you have as a patient is to get up and around the day after surgery.

normal. This is because postoperative pain causes patients to want to remain in bed and to use small, shallow breaths. Diminished breathing effort and poor coughing can cause small parts at the base of the lungs to collapse. Over time, this can cause you to develop a fever, or even pneumonia. You will not damage your incision by walking around as soon as possible or by coughing strongly. To help with pain during coughing, take your pillow, wrap it in front of your abdomen, and hold it firmly against your abdomen while you cough. As physicians, we cannot stress enough the importance of early mobilization after surgery.

After you return home, you can get back to your normal activities relatively quickly. However, you should avoid straining or lifting heavy objects for at least 6 weeks. Take advantage of this situation! It is the perfect opportunity to avoid housework and have your spouse and family members pamper you. You can climb stairs and perform simple chores; however, you should not drive for about 2 weeks after surgery. During this time, you will able to shower and get your incision wet. You can wash it with soapy water and even get the staples wet if they are still in place. However, you should not take baths or go in a swimming pool or hot tub because of the risk of infection.

The scar that results from most abdominal colon operations runs up and down around the **umbilicus** (belly button) in the middle of the belly and is usually about 10 to 15 centimeters long. Most will heal with just a thin scar; however, some groups of people, especially African Americans, can develop a large, thick, hypertrophic (enlarged) scar called a "keloid." The best predictor of how your scar may look is the appearance of other healed scars you might have.

Umbilicus
Belly button.

Pati's Comment:

An incision is sewn in place both inside and out. Your body will let you know when you are overdoing it, trust me. When you get up, press a pillow against your abdomen and slowly swing your legs to the side of the bed. The nurses told me to push the PCA button before I got out of bed; staying ahead of the pain helped. I must have looked like I was 100 years old the first few times I walked all hunched over, but I was able to stand up straight again pretty soon. Yes, it is painful at first, but you will be surprised how fast you heal.

41. How can I get by without part of my colon? What kinds of food can't I eat after surgery?

Although a segment of your colon is removed during surgery, the remaining large intestine is usually able to compensate easily. In the immediate postoperative period, however, you may suffer from diarrhea and increased bowel movements. This is entirely normal. It may take several months before the colon can adequately adapt to the trauma caused by surgery. During this time, it may be helpful to change your diet to a low-residue, low-fiber diet to reduce the bulk that goes into the colon. Table 6 lists some low-fiber dietary recommendations. Several months after surgery, it is unlikely that you will notice any change in bowel habits from your preoperative levels after a standard colectomy.

It may be helpful to change your diet to a low-residue, low-fiber diet.

Kate's Comment:

After each of my surgeries, it has taken time for my bowels to return to a manageable function. Even today, some foods will cause frequent or loose stools, and I usually have small, formed bowel movements several times a day. However, I am able to eat a lot of salads, fruit, and crisp-cooked vegetables. I have a whole grain cereal for breakfast each day. That and a hot cup of coffee help empty my bowels in the morning and avoid urgency or accidents during the day. I limit meat, particularly with fat or gravy, which tends to cause diarrhea with an urgent need to find a bathroom. Greasy or very spicy food will do the same thing.

Table 6 Post-operative diet recommendations

- Breads, grains, carbohydrates: DO EAT: Refined breads, white breads, rolls, biscuits, muffins, waffles, pancakes, refined cereals (like puffed rice, corn flakes), white rice, sweet potato, pastas. AVOID: Whole grains, stone ground, pumpernickel, rye breads, bran or granola cereals, whole grain crackers, corn bread, corn muffins, barley, brown and wild rice.
- Meats/proteins: DO EAT: Ground and well-cooked meats, fish, poultry, eggs, tofu, smooth peanut butter. AVOID: Tough fibrous meats, fried meats and eggs, legumes (e.g., dried beans, kidney, navy, lima, black), crunchy peanut butter.
- Fruits: DO EAT: Canned and cooked fruits, applesauce, banana, cantaloupe, honeydew, nectarine, papaya, peach, plum, watermelon. AVOID: Fruits with skin and seeds, all dried fruits, juice with pulp.
- Vegetables: DO EAT: Most vegetables without seeds, canned vegetables, cucumber, green pepper, spinach, squash, pumpkin. AVOID: Lima beans, green peas, broccoli, parsnips, corn.
- Fats: DO EAT: Margarine, butter, mayonnaise, vegetable oils, salad dressing, plain cakes, cookies, sorbet, pudding, custard, jelly, ice cream, frozen yogurt. AVOID: Nuts, seeds, popcorn, potato chips, raisins, chocolate, coconut, pickles, olives.
- Dairy Products: Most are allowed, but avoid highly flavored cheese.

Because I have had several bowel obstructions, I try to eat only foods that can be chewed well, avoiding tough meat, celery, and most raw vegetables. Popcorn, which I still yearn for, causes serious problems, so I can't eat it at all.

Removal of the rectum, however, presents problems that are different than those occurring in a standard colon resection. Because the rectum is a reservoir for stool before defecation, its removal has a greater effect on lifestyle. Symptoms of increased bowel frequency and urgency are common and usually do not return to preoperative levels. The impact of rectal surgery is discussed in Question 44.

42. What is laparoscopic surgery? Can it be used to treat colon cancer?

Laparoscopic surgery is an example of "minimally invasive surgery." Instead of having a long abdominal incision, during laparoscopic surgery special instruments are used so that major surgery can be performed through several small skin incisions. Since the late 1980s, laparoscopic techniques have become the standard of care for certain operations, such as gallbladder removal and repair of esophageal acid reflux.

In the laparoscopic technique, a small 1-cmcmcm curved incision is made below the umbilicus (belly button), and a tube (trocar) is penetrated through the abdominal wall. Carbon dioxide gas is then blown through the trocar, which expands the abdomen like a balloon, allowing room to manipulate the internal organs. A long, narrow camera is placed through the trocar into the abdominal cavity, displaying a magnified view of the internal organs on television monitors in the operating room. Three to four additional trocars are then placed through separate, small (5- to 10-m) incisions in the abdominal wall. By using specialized instruments that pass through the trocars, surgery that normally requires a large incision can be performed inside the abdomen. For example, the gallbladder can be removed or a piece of bowel can be resected through a very small incision. At the end of the procedure, a slightly larger incision measuring 3 to 6 centimeters is made to remove the portion of colon from inside the abdominal cavity. Sometimes this incision can be hidden below the belt line.

Laparoscopic surgery is a field in constant flux, where improvements in technique are the norm. For example, surgeons can now place a single hand inside the abdomen through a smaller incision to help with the laparoscopic surgery. In some institutions, mechanical robots substitute for human assistants. There are many ways to perform laparoscopic colon surgery. Common to all of these techniques is that they use a smaller incision than open surgery.

The main advantage of laparoscopic surgery is that there is less pain afterwards. Most postoperative pain results from the long abdominal incision and the stretching of the abdominal muscles during open surgical procedures. Because smaller incisions are made and because the surgery is performed within the abdomen, there is less pain with laparoscopic surgery. In general, patients use less pain medication and get out of bed earlier in their hospitalization. Their bowel function returns to normal more quickly, and there may be fewer respiratory complications in certain patients. Cosmetically, the incisions are much smaller, so scars are less visible, and many scars can be hidden in skin folds or below the bikini line. Hospital stays are generally about a day shorter than those with open surgery. Some surgeons believe that fewer adhesions form after laparoscopic surgery, which might mean a lower risk of a small bowel obstruction later, however, this has not yet been proven. Clearly, laparoscopic surgery offers benefit, but there are some limitations to this technique when it is applied to colon resection.

Technically, a laparoscopic colectomy is more difficult to complete than an open colectomy. Laparoscopic techniques are harder to master, and there is the risk for more complications by less experienced surgeons. These operations also take more time to complete and therefore require longer periods of general anesthesia. Unfortunately, prolonged anesthesia can have adverse effects on fragile patients with multiple medical problems. Finally, the surgeon has a greater ability to feel with his or her hands during open surgery, and this ability is limited with laparoscopic techniques. So although laparoscopic surgery has become the standard of care for gallbladder surgery, it is not yet quite the standard for colon surgery.

Laparoscopic surgery is accepted for the management of benign colonic disease like diverticulitis, but it is not widely used in cancer surgery. Because laparoscopic surgery is technically more difficult to perform, there is the fear that surgeons with less experience will perform inadequate oncologic resections (surgical re-movals), leading to worse long-term outcomes. Others believe that because the abdomen is inflated with gas, tumor cells could be spread throughout the abdomen during laparoscopic surgery. Theoretically, these dropped cells could grow, causing metastases at the sites of trocar insertion or even throughout the abdomen.

For these reasons, the use of laparoscopic surgery for colon cancer was tested in a national research trial that compared laparoscopic colon cancer resection with conventional open colon resection. The study was performed by many surgeons at multiple hospitals throughout the United States. The results of this trial were recently published. What this trial showed is that when performed by skilled surgeons, overall survival was the same whether you had an open resection or a laparoscopic resection.

So in general, cancers of the colon can be removed laparoscopically with smaller incisions and in general with a 1 day shorter hospital stay. However, it is important to remember that because of technical issues not all cancers will be able to be removed by laparoscopic methods. If you would like to have laparoscopic surgery instead of the traditional open surgery, you will need to find a surgeon skilled in this technique and find out if you are a candidate.

43. Can I have laser surgery for my colorectal cancer?

Many patients want "laser surgery" for their colorectal cancer. A laser utilizes a high-energy beam of light to burn and cauterize (destroy) tissue. Lasers are commonly used to remove perianal warts and occasionally used to burn through obstructing rectal cancers. Unfortunately, however, laser surgery for colon cancer does not exist. People often confuse laser surgery with laparoscopic surgery.

44. What are the treatment options for rectal cancer—are they different from colon cancer? Do I need to have surgery?

Rectal surgery presents different problems than colon surgery for several reasons. Although the colon moves freely about inside the abdomen, the rectum lies deep within the pelvis and is attached to the backbone and the pelvic sidewalls. Removal of the rectum (**proctectomy**) is technically more difficult, and more complications occur with this surgery than with colon surgery. The rectum lies next to important structures inside the pelvis, including the major blood vessels to the legs; the ureters, which carry urine from the kidneys to the bladder; the prostate; the bladder; and the vagina. By working inside the closed space of the pelvis, there is the possibility of injuring these organs during surgery. Additionally, the nerves responsible for normal urinary function and normal sexual function are close to the rectum. Damage to these nerves can cause urinary and sexual problems. Reconnecting the colon to the lower rectum or anal canal can be difficult in obese patients or in those with a narrow pelvis. Because of the technical difficulties of these operations, with proctectomy there is more tumor recurrence in the pelvis than with colectomy.

Proctectomy
Surgical removal of the rectum.

Another reason rectal surgery is different from colon surgery is that the functions of these two organs are radically different. The colon's ability to absorb fluid is very redundant, meaning that if a section is removed, another section can take over its role. The rectum, on the other hand, stores feces and has a crucial role in our ability to hold the feces inside until a socially appropriate time. Its function cannot be easily replaced, and in most cases, bowel function will never return to normal preoperative levels after rectal surgery. Finally, in advanced cases of rectal cancer, the anal sphincter muscles, which control our continence, are removed during radical surgery. With these muscles removed, the bowel cannot be reconnected and a permanent stoma may be necessary. For these reasons, the details of rectal surgery are discussed separately.

As with tumors of the colon, surgical removal is essentially the only cure for rectal cancer. The segment of rectum containing the tumor must be removed, including the fatty tissue surrounding the blood vessels that supply the colon and the nearby lymph nodes. Additionally, some normal tissue around the tumor must be removed to reduce the risk that the tumor will return. The surgical approaches for rectal cancer vary between limited excisions for small cancerous polyps versus large, radical abdominal approaches for more advanced tumors. Operations that maintain the anal sphincter and avoid a colostomy are called "sphincter-saving" procedures. Examples of this include anterior resections, low anterior resections, and **transanal excisions**. When the sphincter cannot be saved, an **abdominoperineal resection** is necessary. This resection removes the anal sphincter and therefore requires a permanent colostomy. The treatment options for rectal cancer are described below.

Transanal excision

Sphincter-saving technique for removal of small tumors of the lower rectum.

Abdominal resection

Surgical removal of the anus, the rectum, and the surrounding muscles of the anal canal.

Anterior Resection (AR): In an anterior resection, tumors high up in the rectum are removed through an incision in the lower abdomen. The upper rectum and lower part of the colon are removed, and then the ends are reconnected.

Low Anterior Resection (LAR): A low anterior resection is used for tumors of the mid- and lower rectum. As in an anterior resection, the bowel is approached through an incision in the lower abdomen. More tissue is removed in this procedure, including most of the rectum and its entire mesentery (the mesorectum) down to the muscles of the anal sphincter. This **total mesorectal excision** (TME) is the current standard of care for very low tumors and has the lowest rate of tumor recurrence inside the pelvis. The colon is then joined to the lowest portion of the rectum or the anal canal (colo-anal anastamosis). Because a permanent colostomy is not required, this operation is considered to be a sphincter-saving procedure. However, a temporary ileostomy (a loop of small bowel brought out to the skin) may be necessary to protect this anastomosis during the healing period (see Question 46).

Total mesorectal excision (TME)

Surgical removal of most of the rectum and its entire mesentery.

Abdominoperineal Resection (APR): Abdominoperineal resection or APR has historically been the standard of care for tumors of the lower rectum. Two incisions are made, one through the abdomen and the second incision around the anus in the **perineum** (the perineum is the area of the body surrounding the anus and genital structures). During an APR, the anus, the rectum, and the surrounding muscles of the anal canal are entirely removed. Because the muscles of the anal sphincter are removed, bowel continuity cannot be restored, and a permanent colostomy is necessary after APR.

Perineum
The area of the body around the anus and genital structures.

Recently, low rectal cancers that would normally have required an APR have increasingly been treated with sphincter-saving procedures that avoid a permanent colostomy. The main reason for the switch has been the use of new circular surgical staplers that have simplified the procedure. Additionally, smaller tumors of the lower rectum are removed through the anus (see next section). Therefore, the APR is now limited to large tumors that lie very low down in the rectum and affect the muscles of the anal sphincter. Each year, the number of APRs performed in the United States decreases and probably accounts for less than 15% of rectal cancer operations. Sphincter-saving procedures can be substituted for APRs in many cases because they offer the same life expectancy and do not require colostomy.

Transanal Excision (TAE): Transanal excision is used for small tumors of the lower rectum that would normally require an APR. Like a low anterior resection, transanal excision does not require a colostomy and is a sphincter-saving surgery. Rather than completely removing the rectum, the surgeon removes these tumors from the wall of the rectum by operating through the anus. The section of rectum containing the tumor is removed, and sutures are used to close the area. However, because only part of the rectal wall is removed, the nearby lymph nodes are left behind. If these nodes contain microscopic cancer cells, they can be a source for recurrent cancer. For this reason, only smaller, less aggressive tumors are candidates for this surgery.

Some patients object to the idea of rectal surgery, fearing loss of bowel control and the embarrassment of dealing with even a temporary ostomy (see Question 46). However, there is no cure for most rectal cancers other than surgery. Less invasive procedures, such as destruction of the tissue using electric current, laser surgery, or localized radiation therapy, have a limited role in very select circumstances, but in general they cannot cure most rectal cancer.

There is no cure for most rectal cancers other than surgery.

45. I have read about reconstruction after rectal surgery with a colonic J-pouch. What is that?

Bowel function after the rectum is removed never returns to normal because the body has no place to hold stool at the end of the colon. A J-pouch serves as an "imitation rectum" and therefore improves postoperative bowel function.

During a standard low anterior resection with a total mesorectal excision, almost the entire rectum is removed and is replaced by the normal colon, which is attached to the very low rectum or the anal canal. Because the normal colon is narrower and cannot expand as well as the rectum, it cannot hold stool as well as the rectum. Patients have more daily bowel movements, as well as bowel "urgency," which means that once they feel they need to move their bowels, they need a bathroom quickly to avoid incontinence. It is common for these patients to move their bowels 7 or 8 times a day in the first months after surgery. Luckily, these symptoms improve over time as the large bowel compensates. It stretches and thickens, beginning to simulate the previous rectum. After about 2 years, the adjustment period is completed. Patients still move their bowels 3 or 4 times a day and have bowel urgency, however, these symptoms will have improved markedly since surgery. Changes in diet and supplementation with bulk agents, like Metamucil, can significantly help even out bowel activity.

In an attempt to solve this problem , surgeons designed a pouch from the descending colon that imitates the function of the rectum. In this procedure, the end of the colon is looped back on itself, looking like a letter "J". The bowel is then stapled together, creating a pouch about 5 or 6 centimeters long. The pouch thereby imitates the reservoir that is normally created by the rectum. It has a larger capacity than a straight bowel section and expands to store more feces. A novel idea, the colonic J-pouch has been quite successful in improving bowel function after proctectomy. However, bowel function never returns to exactly the way it was before surgery. What a pouch does is allow the patient to reach a stable bowel pattern more quickly. Instead of the typical 2 years that it takes to have stable bowel function, this can be achieved in 3 months with a J-pouch.

Although a J-pouch is generally better than a straight section of bowel under routine circumstances, unfortunately not everyone is a candidate for a pouch. Occasionally the descending colon is too short to reach into the pelvis and also create a pouch. This problem is more common in men than in women because the pelvis tends to be narrower in men. The final decision regarding pouch placement will be made during surgery by your surgeon, however, most patients are able to have one constructed. Most of the time, surgeons will place a temporary ileostomy to protect the pouch and the bowel reconnection until healing is complete.

46. What is an ostomy or stoma?

Everyone seems to know at least one person with a "bag," and so has some idea of what a stoma is. We will try to clarify exactly what it is and clear up some misconceptions. A stoma is simply a loop of intestine that is brought out through the abdominal wall. In this way, intestinal contents drain into a plastic bag that is taped to the skin of the stomach. A stoma can be created either from small bowel (ileostomy) or from large bowel (colostomy).

A stoma is necessary when it is impossible or unsafe to restore bowel continuity during surgery.

The material that drains from an ileostomy is a greenish, acidic liquid similar to bile. Colostomy (large bowel) output is more solid and is similar to normal feces. A stoma can be temporary and can be used to divert intestinal flow for a period of time, or it can be permanent. A stoma is necessary when it is impossible or unsafe to restore bowel continuity during surgery. There are three reasons that a stoma is necessary during routine colorectal cancer surgery.

1. APR: Because the anal sphincter is removed during APR, a colostomy is required. It is not possible to reconnect the colon to the anus after the anal sphincter is removed, because waste would flow out without control. A colostomy after APR is permanent; it is not reversible.
2. Protective diversion: Placement of an ileostomy is common after low anterior resection with reconnection of the bowel to the low rectum or anus. This procedure reduces complications after surgery. The ileostomy is temporary and will be reversed about 3 months after the initial surgery or after postoperative chemotherapy is completed.
3. Colonic obstruction/fecal contamination: An advanced colon cancer can grow so large that it obstructs the normal flow of feces. When the large bowel becomes completely obstructed, the abdomen expands and can cause nausea and vomiting; this condition can be life-threatening. In these cases, immediate surgery is necessary to remove the cancer and decompress the obstructed bowel. Because the bowel is swollen with obstructed feces, reconnecting the bowel would be unsafe. The risk of postoperative leakage is very high, so a colostomy is required. In these instances, the colostomy is usually temporary, and many can be reversed after a few months of recuperation.

47. What are the complications of having a stoma?

In general, stomas are very well tolerated. With adjustments in diet and lifestyle, most patients lead normal lives after the stoma is created. The most common problem caused by a stoma is skin irritation from an ill-fitting bag. This problem is more common with ileostomies because they tend to have a more liquid material than a colostomy. With a combination of different faceplates, adhesives, and skin protectants, however, these problems can be remedied. Your ostomy nurse will be crucial in selecting a system that works for you.

Over time, changes in your body can result in ostomy problems. The surrounding muscle can weaken, allowing the small bowel to penetrate through the abdominal wall (**hernia**). Although the resulting bulge can be unattractive, in general, these hernias are not dangerous and are not cause for alarm. Unfortunately, hernias can recur even after they are repaired, but newer techniques for repair are common. Another complication can arise if the stoma opening becomes too large. In these cases, several inches of bowel can push out of the stoma, which can be frightening to look at. This is called a prolapse. Although this condition causes little medical problem, surgery is necessary to remove the excess bowel.

Hernia
A loop of bowel or an organ that protrudes through an abnormal opening in the body.

48. Will I need a colostomy?

The first question after being diagnosed with rectal cancer is "Will I need a bag?" and rightfully so. A colostomy is a life-altering adjustment both physically and emotionally. Hopefully, Questions 46 and 47 have adequately explained the nature of an ostomy. People generally lead a normal life with these appliances. Luckily, with improvements in surgical technique and technology, fewer colostomies are being performed every year. Many tumors that required APR in the past are now removed using sphincter-saving approaches. These procedures are possible because they provide a cure that is equivalent to that provided by APR. Keep in mind that the primary goal is your survival. Thousands of people lead long lives with a permanent colostomy, having been cured of their rectal cancer, and with assistance from the medical team and other supports, they learn how to successfully live life with an ostomy (see Part 5, Changes Cancer Brings).

When first diagnosed with rectal cancer, you may be overwhelmed by the news and the thought of needing a permanent colostomy. We will try to simplify this decision process in the next few questions. Everything is dependent on whether the muscles of the anal sphincter can be saved. Remember, if these are removed, a permanent colostomy is required. The ability of your surgeon to perform a "sphincter-sparing" procedure is dependent on two factors: tumor location and tumor stage. You should be able to discuss these issues with your surgeon.

1. Tumor location: Cancers that are very low in the rectum and abut the anal sphincter may not be removable with a low anterior resection. These tumors require either an APR or a transanal excision (surgery performed through the anus).
2. Tumor stage: Only very early stage, favorable tumors are suitable for transanal excision. Large, aggressive tumors that have a high risk for spread to the lymph nodes are not candidates for transanal excision.

Tumor location and tumor stage determine the kind of surgery that is appropriate. Ask your surgeon these two important questions: Can my tumor be removed with a transanal approach or will I need an abdominal operation (see Question 49)? If I need an abdominal operation, can the sphincter be saved or will I need a permanent colostomy (see Question 50)?

49. Can my tumor be removed with a transanal approach or will I need an open surgery?

Transanal excision (TAE, surgery performed through the anus) is a good treatment for very select rectal cancers for several reasons. First, it is a sphincter-saving procedure that enables the patient to maintain bowel control and avoid having a permanent colostomy. Second, because it is performed through the anus and without an abdominal incision, it is less invasive and has a lower risk of complications than an open procedure.

Unfortunately, transanal excision is not for everyone. Because transanal excision is performed through the anal canal, only small tumors that are low down in the rectum can be removed—it is just not possible to remove large tumors that are high up in the rectum. These require an abdominal operation.

In addition, unlike the techniques of an abdominal rectal removal, nearby lymph nodes are not removed with a transanal approach. If these nodes contain cancerous deposits and are not surgically removed, the tumor will continue to grow and eventually recur inside the pelvis. Tumors that are at high risk for spread to the local lymph nodes are therefore not candidates for transanal excision. The risk of lymph node spread is related to the size of the tumor and the depth of the tumor at presentation. The larger the size, the more locally advanced the tumor, and the higher the risk of lymph node spread (see Question 28 for explanation of tumor grading and staging).

- T0: Limited to the mucosal lining of the colon, these "in situ" cancers are ideal candidates for transanal excision. They present absolutely no risk for lymph node spread, and local removal will cure them.
- T1: In general, T1 lesions are good candidates for transanal excision. The risk of lymph node spread is

only 5% to 10% in carefully selected T1 tumors. However, even among T1 tumors, some lesions have adverse microscopic characteristics that suggest a higher chance of spread to adjacent lymph nodes. These aggressive cancers are not reliably treated with transanal excision, and more radical surgery is necessary.
- T2/T3: T2 and T3 lesions invade the muscle of the rectal wall and present a 20% to 50% chance for lymph node spread. These cancers are therefore not candidates for transanal excision and require a radical approach.

It is important to know the tumor size, as well as depth of penetration before surgery, to help identify patients who can undergo transanal excision. There are many ways to determine the preoperative depth of a rectal cancer, however, endorectal ultrasound is the gold standard (see Question 51). Endorectal ultrasound can accurately determine the extent of tumor invasion and can even suggest the presence of abnormal lymph nodes. It is extremely useful in identifying candidates for TAE.

50. My tumor cannot be removed by transanal excision and requires an open surgery. Can I still have sphincter-saving surgery?

This is the second issue to be considered when determining the need for a permanent colostomy. Your surgeon has determined that transanal excision is not possible and that you therefore need an abdominal operation. This [Abdominal surgery] does not mean you require a permanent colostomy. Abdominal approaches include low anterior resection (LAR, a sphincter-saving procedure) and abdominoperineal resection (APR, removal of the muscles of the anal canal, requiring a permanent colostomy). In properly selected patients, life expect-ancy after LAR is the same as after APR.

[Abdominal surgery] does not mean you require a permanent colostomy.

Whether an LAR can be performed instead of an APR is determined by the location of the tumor within the rectum. Tumors lying a few centimeters or more from the anal canal can be removed with the sphincter-saving LAR procedure; those lying closer to the anal canal cannot generally be removed with an LAR and require a permanent colostomy. Endorectal ultrasound can be very helpful in clarifying the placement of the tumor and its relation to the anal sphincter muscles.

51. How is rectal cancer staged before surgery? Is it really necessary to undergo an ultrasound for rectal cancer?

Accurate preoperative staging of rectal cancer is essential to provide the best therapy and to determine whether sphincter-saving surgery can be performed. Historically, tumors were staged only through physical examination, which depended on the sensitivity of the examining surgeon's index finger. Unfortunately, the accuracy of clinical examination is 60% at best, and enlarged perirectal lymph nodes cannot be detected this way. Radiologic studies, like CT and MRI scanning, are useful additions to the digital rectal examination. However, endorectal ultrasound has become the gold standard for staging rectal cancer before surgery.

Endorectal ultrasound uses sound waves to create a two-dimensional image of the rectum. This illustrates the layers of the bowel wall, allowing the tumor depth to be determined using staging criteria. The examination is not very invasive and can be performed in your doctor's office. The only preparation required is two Fleet® enemas, taken the morning of the procedure. After standard digital rectal examination and proctoscopic exam, the ultrasound probe is passed through the proctoscope into the rectum. A balloon on the tip of the probe is filled with water, and ultrasound images are created by sound waves. The entire examination is completed in only 5 to 10 minutes. Although the proctoscopy is uncomfortable, the procedure is not painful and sedation is not required. Endorectal ultrasound is extremely accurate in predicting tumor depth and identifying suspicious nearby lymph nodes.

In experienced hands, endorectal ultrasound is accurate 80% of the time in staging rectal cancer before surgery. When errors occur, they tend toward overestimating rather than underestimating the stage of the cancer. Therefore, treatment is even more thorough.

Endorectal ultrasound can also detect abnormal lymph nodes around the rectum that may contain cancer. Abnormal nodes appear larger and darker than normal nodes on the ultrasound. In general, the presence of suspicious lymph nodes on ultrasound is an indication for more aggressive treatment. Because some of these enlarged nodes are inflamed (irritated), however, and do not actually contain metastatic cancer, the ultrasound is only about 60% accurate in correctly selecting enlarged nodes that contain metastases. In addition, endorectal ultrasound cannot identify small lymph nodes that contain only microscopic spread.

Finally, the ultrasound can detect a tumor that has spread into the muscles of the anal sphincter. In these cases, sphincter-saving surgery cannot be performed, and APR (total removal of the anus, the rectum, and the surrounding muscles of the anal canal) is required. For all these reasons, endorectal ultrasound should be a standard test in the preoperative evaluation of rectal cancer. It can determine tumor stage and sphincter muscle invasion, which are two important issues in determining which surgical approach should be used.

Other radiologic examinations have been used in preoperative evaluation, including CT and MRI scans. CT scanning is a less precise method of staging tumors of the rectum; however, because it is used to evaluate the liver for metastases (cancer spread) before surgery, it is a routine test during preoperative workup. CT is very good at identifying obvious disease around the rectum—it is extremely accurate at identifying very enlarged lymph nodes or extensive spread into surrounding structures, such as the bladder or prostate. However, it cannot identify the fine layers of the rectum, and therefore cannot give an accurate tumor depth before surgery. MRI scanning, on the other hand, is very good at distinguishing the layers of the rectum when performed with the use of additional specialized equipment. Unfortunately, MRI scanning for rectal cancer has some drawbacks. First, this test needs to be performed at specialized MRI centers. It requires an extra visit and is much more expensive than endorectal ultrasound. In addition, MRI can increase anxiety in some people because it requires lying still in an enclosed space. However, use of relaxation techniques, such as deep breathing, and/or prescriptions to reduce anxiety can help people with anxiety to successfully complete the MRI. Talk to your doctor about your concerns about any procedure so that you can explore these options. And, in spite of the additional cost, MRI is still only as accurate as endorectal ultrasound. Therefore, endorectal ultrasound remains the best, simplest, and least invasive measure for preoperative rectal cancer staging. We believe that every person with a newly diagnosed rectal cancer should undergo preoperative diagnosis with ultrasound.

52. Are the risks of rectal surgery different from the risks of colon surgery?

The risks of proctectomy (removal of the rectum) are the same as those of any abdominal surgery, including the risks posed by anesthesia, the risk of bleeding requiring a blood transfusion, and the risk of postoperative infection (see Question 38). However, unlike colon surgery, there are additional complications that are specific to pelvic surgery and proctectomy. These include **neuropathy**, ureteral injury, and sexual dysfunction.

Neuropathy
Disruption in a nerve's function, sometimes caused by trauma, such as during surgery.

Neuropathy results from trauma to a nerve. During rectal surgery, you are positioned on your back with your legs raised up in stirrups. This is necessary to give your surgeon access to the area being operated on. During this time, your legs are padded and special stockings are placed on them to prevent blood clots from forming. Unfortunately, being in this position for several hours can cause pressure on the nerves of the leg. Every measure is taken to prevent this, however, prolonged pressure can cause leg numbness and weakness after surgery. The good news is that this complication is extremely rare, and the symptoms are almost always temporary; sensation usually returns to normal over a period of several weeks.

During pelvic surgery there is also the risk of damage to the ureters, the structures that carry urine from the kidneys to the bladder. These small, tubular organs run down into the pelvis next to the rectum. When rectal tumors grow very large, they can distort the normal anatomy and may damage the ureters. The risk is greatest in the case of large tumors and recurrent cancers. In these cases, your surgeon may ask to have a **urologist** (a surgeon who specializes in diseases of the urinary tract) place special tubes into the ureters preoperatively, to help the surgeon find them during surgery. In the rare instance that the ureters are injured, they are usually repaired during the surgery without long-term complications. Unnoticed ureteral injuries may be more serious and may have long-term consequences.

Urologist

Surgeon who specializes in diseases of the urinary tract.

Finally, the nerves that lead to the bladder and sexual organs run along the backbone into the pelvis, and wrap around the prostate in men. Every effort is made to spare these nerves during removal of the rectum. But because the rectum is so close to the prostate, injury to these nerves can occur and can result in sexual dysfunction (see Question 62) and urinary retention.

53. Will I need a temporary ostomy after a low anterior resection with a colonic J-pouch?

This is a controversial topic among colorectal surgeons. The answer, however, is usually "yes." In general, when the colon is joined to the anal canal after proctectomy (coloanal anastomosis) with a colonic J-pouch, most surgeons will perform a temporary ileostomy to protect the connection during healing. If a protective ileostomy is not used, even under the best circumstances, a few of these connections will leak, and although a small leak may not cause any symptoms and will go unnoticed, in other cases leaks can cause severe pelvic infection. After a major leak, surgery is required to drain the infection, and in some instances creation of a permanent colostomy may be necessary. In order to avoid this occurrence, at the time of the rectal cancer removal and the sphincter saving procedure a loop of small bowel is brought through the abdominal wall (a loop ileostomy), so that all fecal flow from the bowel exits here. The ileostomy serves to "protect" the surgical connection between the two ends of the reconnected bowel. Although this measure does not prevent a leak, it does reduce the risk that severe abdominal sepsis (severe infection) will occur if a small leak develops.

This ileostomy is only temporary. Your surgeon will wait 2 to 3 months after surgery and then perform a Gastrografin® enema study to evaluate the pouch. If the study shows that healing is complete, your ileostomy can be reversed. Because chemotherapy can affect the body's ability to heal, most surgeons wait until postoperative chemotherapy is completed before they consider reversing the ileostomy. (This can extend your wait to 4 to 6 months after surgery.) Most ileostomies can be reversed with a small incision around the ileostomy itself and do not require a major abdominal incision. The hospital stay after this surgery is usually only 3 to 5 days.

54. Which is better to have, a sphincter-saving operation with coloanal J-pouch or a permanent colostomy?

Although postoperative bowel function and quality of life are important, the most important consideration is your survival. Sphincter-saving surgery should never be a substitute for surgery that could cure you. It must provide a chance of survival and risk of recurrence that is the same as that of radical surgery. Fortunately, multiple studies have confirmed that, when possible, low anterior resection (removal of the rectum down to the muscles of the anal sphincter) is equivalent to APR (total removal of the anus, the rectum, and the surrounding muscles of the anal canal).

Sphincter-saving surgery should never be a substitute for surgery that could cure you.

It seems impossible to believe, therefore, that choosing a colostomy could ever be better than reconnecting the bowel after rectal surgery. However, bowel function after proctectomy (removal of the rectum) with a sphincter-saving procedure never returns to normal preoperative levels. The physiologic activity of the normal rectum is extremely complicated and cannot be replaced, even with a J-pouch. Additionally, surgery involving the anal canal can damage already-weakened muscles of the anal sphincter which can weaken because of changes caused by childbirth in women and from simple aging in older patients. Therefore, patients may suffer from increased bowel frequency, urgency, and incontinence after this type of surgery.

Many professionals have debated the question of quality of life after LAR with a J-pouch connection between the colon and anus. Keep in mind, some people will do anything to avoid a permanent colostomy. They will tolerate increased bowel frequency (3 to 4 times or more during the day, and possibly at night) and irritation around the anus. With this condition, the patient sometimes cannot postpone defecation longer than a few minutes, and often stays constantly near a bathroom because they are afraid of accidents. There may be episodes of leaking of small amounts of gas and liquid, and patients may have to use small pads to prevent staining. Many of these problems are worse in people with a history of previous incontinence (which is common in the elderly). Women who have given birth several times are at risk for hidden anal sphincter damage, which may not become evident until after surgery, showing up as an increased frequency and looseness of bowel movements.

It is hard to quantify these problems. Complaints of urgency, frequency, leakage, and incontinence are subjective (depend on the person's perception) and are compared with the patient's function before surgery. In general, patients who have undergone abdominoperineal resection (APR) with permanent colostomy describe a worsening of self-image and more psychosocial problems associated with the colostomy. However, overall quality of life may actually be better in patients with colostomies because they experience fewer limitations of their daily activities, are less restricted by bowel activity, feel healthier, and get more sleep than patients with coloanal anastomosis.

Your surgeon can give you objective advice. He or she can tell you where the tumor is located, whether an APR is necessary, or whether reconstruction of the bowel is even possible. If reconstruction is possible, however, your final decision is a personal one. If you are already suffering from minor leaking of gas or liquid, then reconstruction is likely not the right option. However, if you are a healthy, motivated patient and can cope with the initial problems that reconnection between the colon and the anus presents, this may be the optimal choice.

55. Where does advanced colorectal-cancer tend to spread?

Colon cancer, like other cancers, spreads in various ways. By growing larger, it spreads into the surrounding tissues. This is not considered metastatic spread. Instead, the initial tumor extends locally beyond its natural location, invading the surrounding organs, including the spleen, pancreas, kidney, and ureter. Rectal tumors, which lie deep inside the pelvis, have less room to spread. They grow and can extend into the prostate, vagina, bladder, or even the bones of the spine. These tumors are labeled T4 lesions.

Cancers that spread beyond the colon usually spread via the lymph node channels and the veins that lead out from the area (Figure 6). Because veins from the colon drain through the liver, 80% of distant metastases are to the liver. Unfortunately, 15% to 25% of patients with colorectal cancer have metastases (Stage IV disease) at the time they are first diagnosed. Because the venous drainage of the lower rectum is different from that of the colon, these tumors also tend to spread to the lungs.

CHEMOTHERAPY: CURRENT PRACTICE AND NEW DEVELOPMENTS

56. What are the other therapies besides surgery?

Although not a cure, chemotherapy is a non-surgical treatment for cancer that helps improve long-term survival. **Acupuncture** and homeopathy may help some patients cope with the side effects of cancer treatment, but only chemotherapy and radiation therapy have been shown to improve survival in patients with colorectal cancer. These techniques are used to improve the outcomes of surgery, and they may be administered either before or after the surgery.

Acupuncture

A Chinese therapy involving the use of thin needles placed in special pressure points on the body.

Chemotherapy (or "chemo") simply means using drugs to treat disease; in this case, cancer. Chemotherapy agents act by limiting cell division, prohibiting DNA replication, and encouraging the body's own immune system to attack malignant cells. In reality, these substances are actually poisons that halt the overall cell growth. They may target cancer cells primarily, but they affect normal cells as well. The ideal cancer drug

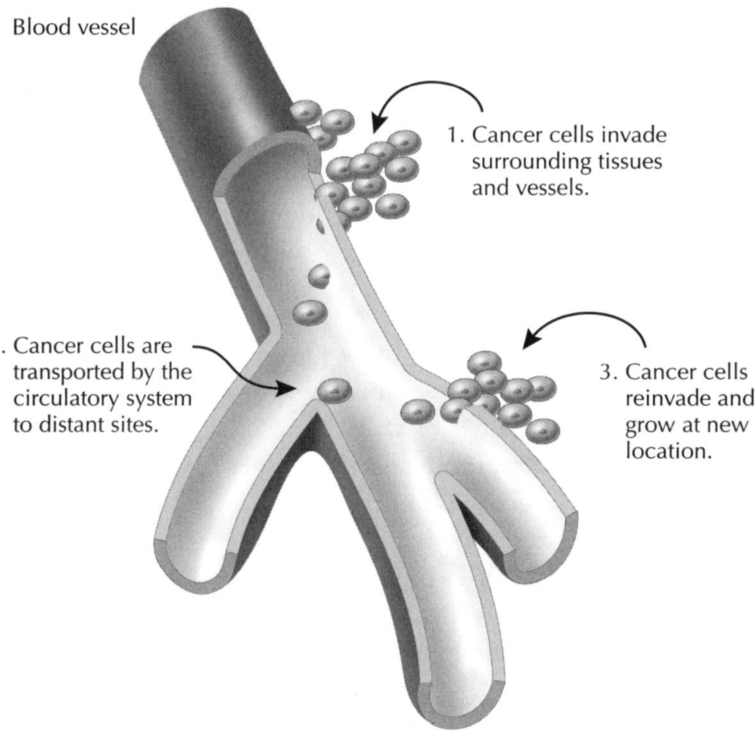

Figure 6 Routes of metastasis.

would isolate only tumor cells and would not harm normal human tissue. Although extensive research continues to try to create these "magic bullets" that attack only cancer cells, current types of chemotherapy are usually not this precise and are toxic to normal cells as well. Because of this, chemotherapy may produce side effects.

Radiation therapy (also called "radiotherapy" or "RT") uses high-energy electromagnetic radiation to treat cancer by damaging the cancer cell's DNA and causing cell death. Radiation therapy is used more commonly in the treatment of rectal cancer to shrink tumors before surgery, to sterilize the area to be operated on, and to prevent local recurrence. Radiation therapy can also be used for pain control with large tumors that invade local structures like bone and nerves. In rare tumors of the anal canal, radiation and chemo-therapy are the primary treatments.

In combination therapy, chemotherapy and radiation therapy can be administered together (combination therapy can also consist of more than one anticancer drug given together). Often, chemotherapy agents are used to sensitize tumor cells and make them more susceptible to radiation treatments. When radiation therapy and chemotherapy are given after surgery, they are called adjuvant therapy, and when they are given before the surgery, they are called **neoadjuvant therapy**. Neoadjuvant techniques have several advantages. Shrinking the tumor before surgery allows for a more complete surgical removal, and often sphincter-saving techniques can be applied. Lower doses of radiation can be given with better effect, and this spares the normal tissues from radiation toxicity. Studies continue to demonstrate excellent results with neoadjuvant techniques for locally advanced rectal cancer (tumors extending beyond the wall of the rectum and/or with involvement of lymph nodes), and they are becoming the standard of care in most institutions.

Neoadjuvant theraphy

Radiation therapy and chemotherapy given before surgery.

57. When should someone receive chemotherapy, and when should someone receive radiation therapy? Are they interchangeable?

Chemotherapy and radiation therapy are techniques that aim to eradicate microscopic cancer cell deposits and hidden tumors that may remain after surgery. Chemotherapy is not a substitute for radiation therapy and vice versa. Each of these treatments has different targets and actions.

Radiation therapy is ideal for use against tumors that are locally advanced (large, with spread through the bowel wall) which pose a high risk for recurring in the original tumor site (local recurrence). The problem of local recurrence is more common in the confined space of the pelvis and is therefore more commonly associated with rectal cancer. Radiation therapy sterilizes the area around the cancer, thereby reducing local recurrence.

Chemotherapy, on the other hand, is used to stop or slow down the progression of cancer. Due to side effects, it is not possible to use radiation treatments on the entire body in order to prevent recurrence. Once a tumor has spread into the lymph nodes, the cancer is considered a systemic disease (affecting the whole body). Although the entire tumor that is visible is removed at surgery, there may be many areas of microscopic disease that are not yet visible, possibly in the liver, lungs, or abdominal cavity. Chemotherapy affects both the tumor and the microscopic disease. It is administered intravenously and distributed throughout the body—and used for the prevention and treatment of cancer recurrence.

The reason chemotherapy is used in conjunction with radiation treatment for rectal cancer is that chemo-therapy sensitizes the rectal cancer cells to the effects of radiation, thus making the cancer more responsive to the radiation therapy.

58. Do all patients with colorectal cancer need adjuvant chemotherapy or radiation therapy?

Chemotherapy and radiation therapy can help patients live with cancer longer, however, they also cause side effects, which in certain cases may present significant problems. For example, some chemotherapy regimens cause severe nausea, loss of appetite, and hair loss. Radiation therapy for rectal cancer can cause diarrhea, infection, and reproductive sterility. It is important to note that most of these side effects are effectively managed with appropriate medication. For these reasons, oncologists and their patients need to carefully evaluate the benefits and risks of chemotherapy and radiotherapy. Like all treatments, the benefits of these therapies must outweigh their side effects.

Benefits of these therapies must outweigh their side effects.

Chemotherapy is considered successful if they can decrease the rate of local recurrence, increase the time between initial surgery and cancer recurrence, and ultimately improve survival.

Colon Cancer: Stage I colon cancers are cured with surgery alone, and chemotherapy does not benefit patients with this stage of disease. Stage III colon cancers, on the other hand, are advanced tumors that already show evidence of spread to local lymph nodes. These cancers are considered "systemic diseases" (throughout the whole body) and are likely to spread even after surgery. Individuals with these cancers are the perfect candidates for chemo-therapy. Some studies have shown that treatment with standard chemotherapy regimens decreases the rate of tumor recurrence from 60% to 40% and increases the 5-year survival from 50% to 60%. In 1990, it was widely agreed that adjuvant chemotherapy should be used for Stage III colon cancer, and this remains the standard of care. Currently, clinical trials are attempting to improve the survival rate after surgery for Stage III colon cancer by evaluating combinations of more advanced chemotherapy and novel molecularly targeted agents which have demonstrated much success for more advanced Stage IV colon cancer.

Controversy surrounds the use of adjuvant therapy in Stage II disease. Stage II cancers are large tumors that have spread through the bowel wall but not yet to the surrounding lymph nodes. Some evidence suggests that survival might be increased in patients with Stage II tumors who receive postoperative chemotherapy and Stage II colon cancer presenting with high risk features (see Question 28) should also be considered for chemotherapy. Stage II colon cancer patients presenting without high risk features may not benefit from chemotherapy. For this reason, the choice to receive chemotherapy for Stage II colon cancer should be an informed decision between the treating oncologist and the patient. Healthy people whose tumors are deemed aggressive may want to opt for systemic chemo-therapy (chemo-therapy given intravenously and dispersed throughout the body). Research and clinical trials for Stage II colon cancer are ongoing.

Stage IV colon cancers have already spread to distant organs, like the liver or the lungs. While some Stage IV colon cancers have a limited pattern of spread to a specific organ and can still be surgically removed for cure in some cases, in general, most patients have more extensive spread of the cancer and surgery is often not recommended. Chemotherapy is palliative (for relief of symptoms) and is the primary treatment for patients with Stage IV colon cancer. Finally, there has been no evidence to suggest that radiation therapy is beneficial in the treatment of primary colon cancer.

Recent findings suggest that select patients with Stage IV colon cancers where the cancer has spread only to the liver have a good chance at longer survival if the patient can become a surgical candidate for resection. A significant portion of the liver can be removed with no negative impact on the function of the liver, as the liver can regenerate. Colon cancer with liver metastases needs to be evaluated carefully by a team of an oncologist and a surgeon who preferably specialize in liver surgery. If the surgeon considers the liver metastasis to be at least partially resectable, then both surgery and chemotherapy would be appropriate. Recent studies have suggested that advanced chemotherapeutic and molecularly targeted agents can render some patients to surgical candidacy if the cancer responds well to the therapy. However, every patient should have an individualized approach which requires both the surgeon and the medical oncologist.

Rectal Cancer: Historically, after surgery for rectal cancer, there is a high likelihood of local recurrence in the pelvis. Large T3 cancers (and those with lymph node spread) recurred about 30% of the time after surgery alone; however, the rate of local recurrence has decreased because of improvements in surgical technique and the use of TME (removal of the rectum down to the muscles of the anal sphincter and its attached mesentery; see Question 44). But the recent use of perioperative radiation therapy has had the greatest impact on the treatment of locally advanced rectal cancer (i.e., cancer that has spread into nearby tissues). With the combination of improved surgical technique and adjuvant radiation therapy, the risk of local recurrence in advanced cancers is now less than half of what it once was, or about 10%.

Unfortunately, radiation therapy alone to the pelvis does not treat the systemic spread (i.e., spread throughout the body) of cancer and therefore has not been conclusively shown to increase long-term survival after rectal surgery. However, when radiation therapy was combined with chemotherapy (combination therapy), local recurrences decreased and long-term survival increased in patients with advanced tumors. Combination therapy has been the standard of care for Stage II and Stage III rectal cancer for many years.

As in Stage I colon cancer, adjuvant therapies have not been helpful in Stage I rectal cancer. Stage IV rectal cancers present a difficult management problem that, in a very small number of cases, can still be approached with the intent to cure. Generally, though, they are managed by palliative chemotherapy (for symptom relief and not for cure).

59. What exactly is radiation therapy?

Radiation therapy uses high-dose electromagnetic radiation to treat malignant tumors. Like chemotherapy drugs, high doses of radiation cause injury to the cell. The goal of radiation therapy can be either destroying the tumor or, in the case of patients with extensive cancer spread, symptom relief. Most commonly, it is delivered through the skin (external-beam radiation therapy), but radiation can also be delivered during surgery.

The radiation beam is focused onto the region in the body containing the tumor. The higher the administered dose, the more tumor cells are killed. But because normal cells are also killed, maximum dosages are limited by the effects of the radiation on nearby organs. Unfortunately, all tissues within the dosage field receive the same levels of radiation. For example, during radiation therapy to the rectum, the radiation passes through skin, muscle, bone, bladder, and sexual organs before reaching the rectum. All these organs are at risk for radiation damage as the treatment dose increases. Radiation therapy is therefore adjusted to maximize cancer killing while minimizing effects on nearby tissue. The total dose administered and the area that will receive treatment are the variables adjusted by the radiation oncologist.

Because certain cell types are more susceptible to radiation than others, some cancers are better treated with radiation therapy. This also means that sensitive organs in the radiation fields (areas that receive the radiation) are more susceptible to radiation damage. Organs like the eye, spinal cord, and kidney are easily damaged by radiation,. Special care must be taken to minimize radiation exposure to these organs. One way to reduce radiation toxicity is by dividing the total radiation doses into several smaller amounts over a longer period of time. This allows for maximal tumor killing with minimal toxicity to adjacent tissues—normal cells are spared, while rapidly dividing cancer cells are attacked. Even with these techniques, though, the amount of radiation that can be administered safely before severe tissue damage occurs is still limited.

Although radiation is an excellent adjuvant therapy, it is not a substitute for surgery. Radiation therapy decreases the risk of local recurrence after radical surgery, but it cannot replace the need for surgery. It also cannot correct for poor surgical decision making. For example, transanal excision of a T2 or T3 lesion is not recommended, because of the high risk of lymph node spread and, therefore, of local recurrence. Radiation therapy plus transanal excision for advanced tumors still leads to excessively high recurrence and poor outcomes, so it's not a good choice. Although it may allow for the sphincter to be preserved and avoid the need for a colostomy, this treatment does not provide the same chance for survival as radical resection. Radiation therapy should not be used as a substitute for adequate surgical treatment.

Although radiation is an excellent adjuvant therapy, it is not a substitute for surgery.

60. Is radiation therapy given before or after surgery?

This is a common question nowadays, because radiation therapy is often administered before rather than after surgery, which may seem strange. It is well understood that radiation therapy in conjunction with good surgical treatment (total mesorectal excision—the removal of the rectum down to the muscles of the anal sphincter, with removal of its attached mesentery) of rectal cancer reduces the chances of local recurrence in patients with locally advanced tumors. The com-bination of radiation therapy and chemotherapy decreases local recurrence and increases long-term survival. For this reason, postoperative chemotherapy and radiation (chemoradiation) treatment has been the standard of care for many years and is still used in many institutions. In these cases, your physician will wait 4 to 6 weeks after surgery so that you will have time to recover adequately. You should then be able to receive standard chemoradiation treatments.

So why should radiation be given before surgery rather than after? There are several reasons. First of all, if chemoradiation is given before surgery, the abnormal tissue, the cancer-containing rectum, will receive the brunt of the treatment. After surgery, the rectum is removed and is often replaced with a colonic J-pouch. If radiation is administered then, all the energy will be directed toward the new pouch, which would worsen the patient's already-compromised bowel function. Toxicity is therefore less with preoperative treatment than with postoperative treatment.

Another reason to have chemoradiation therapy before surgery is that it can shrink the tumor and make surgery easier. Tumors that might have required an APR (total removal of the anus, rectum, and surrounding muscles of the anal canal) because of their closeness to the anal sphincter may instead shrink enough to be removed with a sphincter-saving procedure. This is a considerable advantage.

Chemoradiation therapy is also effective in T3 tumors of the rectum that invade through the rectal wall and in tumors that have spread to the lymph nodes. It is usually not recommended in other situations. Endorectal ultrasound can help determine whether the tumor is a T3 tumor and should be treated by chemoradiation therapy. This would mean that people who would not be helped by chemoradiation therapy would not receive it and its side effects unnecessarily.

Preoperative chemoradiation therapy has therefore become the standard of care for patients who we think will benefit from it. However, the only way to identify these patients before surgery is to know the stage of tumor at the time of presentation.

Pati's Comment:

Your team of doctors will determine whether radiation is best given before or after surgery for you. In my case, it was given prior to surgery in hopes of reducing the tumor to avoid a colostomy. By the time of surgery, all that was left was an ulcer where the tumor had been.

61. How is radiation therapy administered and how often? Will I need to be hospitalized for treatment?

Radiation therapy is given commonly in conjunction with chemotherapy for the preoperative treatment of locally advanced rectal cancer. If endorectal ultrasound reveals that you have a deeply invasive rectal cancer, you will be referred to both a radiation oncologist and a medical oncologist for treatment. The radiation oncologist will individualize your radiation therapy, and the medical oncologist will coordinate your chemotherapy by selecting the right medications, the right quantity, and the best way of administering it. Because most standard treatments combine chemo and RT, these two doctors will work closely together to administer treatment.

Simulation

The initial consultation with your radiation oncologist where the exact fields for your radiation will be created.

Radiation treatments begin first with a **simulation** in which your doctor decides which areas of your body will undergo the treatment. You will be given barium (a contrast substance that can be seen on an x-ray) by mouth and through your rectum. Small, permanent ink tattoos may be placed on your skin so that future treatments can be directed in the exact same place each time you have RT.

The standard radiation therapy for rectal cancer lasts 5 weeks. You will come every day, Monday to Friday, for treatments. Although the actual treatment itself only lasts about 15 minutes, you should figure on spending about an hour at the hospital. Do not worry—there is absolutely no pain during the actual administration of radiation treatments. Chemotherapy, although administered in a different outpatient area, is given with radiation.

Pati's Comment:

My radiation oncologist's treatment rooms were actually located in the hospital; I went Monday through Friday for a total of 27 sessions. I also had chemo the first and last 3 days of radiation, so I just walked to the oncologist's office in the building next door. Radiation only took about 5 minutes. The technicians went out of their way to minimize embarrassment, and I was covered with a sheet. The machine made a buzzing noise, so I visualized an angry swarm of bees, stinging the heck out of the cancer. It didn't hurt a bit, the sound just made me think of bees—it made the time pass faster, and felt I was "doing my part."

62. What are the side effects of radiation therapy? Will I be able to have children after treatment?

The side effects of radiation therapy result from damage to other organs that fall inside the radiation field (the area that receives the radiation). The organs in which most toxicity occurs include the bladder, bones of the pelvis, reproductive organs, and small bowel. Side effects include diarrhea, low blood counts, and skin changes.

Short-Term Side Effects

Pati's Comment:

I had a pretty easy time with radiation until the last 2 weeks. At the first sign of skin redness, I was given an aloe vera gel to use; when bowel movements increased, I was given a low residue diet to help decrease these. I really feel this helped me avoid diarrhea during radiation. I used a sitz bath a few times a day, which really soothed my skin. My hemorrhoids flared up, but suppositories with cortisone helped immensely. I met weekly with my radiology oncologist and a dietitian; they closely monitored my labs and weight. I was a little fatigued, but just took it easy and listened to my body.

The short-term side effects begin about 1 to 2 weeks after therapy begins and last until about 1 or 2 weeks after therapy is completed. Most of these can be controlled by simple changes in daily activity and over-the-counter medications. However, they require careful monitoring and care to prevent more serious complications from occurring. Overall, most patients tolerate radiation therapy very well and can continue working on a part-time basis. However, 15% to 20% of patients require brief treatment breaks because of worsening symptoms, and about 5% may actually require a brief hospitalization.

Diarrhea: The most common side effect of radiation therapy for rectal cancer is diarrhea caused by the effects of combined radiation and chemotherapy on the bowel. It is important that you continue to drink lots of fluids during this time so that you don't get too dehydrated from the diarrhea. You should also avoid certain types of food that can make the diarrhea worse, such as foods high in fat or fiber. In most instances, diarrhea can be controlled with diet and medications prescribed by your doctor; however, if the side effects are too severe, you may need to take a break from treatment.

Bone Marrow Suppression: Because the bones of the pelvis are a major site of blood cell production, you may have a decreased white blood cell count and platelet count during radiation therapy. White blood cells are important in fighting infection, so you may be at slightly more risk for infection during therapy. Although you should not avoid contact with friends and family, use good judgment in visiting people who have colds or other infections. Platelets are responsible for blood clotting after cuts and scrapes. Although it is very rare for platelet counts to drop too low, bleeding gums and nosebleeds may be signs of a falling platelet count. Your doctor will take blood tests routinely during your treatment to check these levels. If they drop dangerously low, a treatment pause may be necessary to allow them to replenish. Generally, blood counts return to normal levels after therapy is over.

Bladder: Radiation can damage the bladder, causing frequent urination, urinary urgency, and burning with urination. You should continue to drink more liquids during therapy to reduce your risk of these problems. Medications are available to help treat the bladder spasms that sometimes result from radiation therapy.

Skin: Radiation therapy causes redness and irritation of the skin, and hair in the areas receiving radiation will fall out. Because therapy is aimed at the rectum, the perianal skin is easily irritated. Applying a simple moisturizing lotion such as Aquaphor® to the affected area alone (not the entire area) can be very helpful. You should avoid scented and perfumed soaps, which can irritate the skin. Although the areas receiving radiation therapy for rectal cancer are often hidden, you should still avoid prolonged exposure to the sun.

Fatigue is a common symptom during radiation therapy.

Fatigue: Fatigue is a common symptom during radiation therapy and can have many causes, however, many of these are treatable. First of all, make sure you are getting enough good sleep. See your doctor if persistent insomnia or severe anxiety are limiting your sleep (see Part 5 of this book,

Changes Cancer Brings, to learn more about coping and ways to reduce anxiety). Don't feel bad about taking naps during the day, if necessary. Solicit the help of friends or family to finish chores. Continue to exercise and work as much as you can, but don't overdo it.

LONG-TERM SIDE EFFECTS

Women

The reproductive organs, including the vagina, uterus, and ovaries, lie within the areas undergoing radiation therapy and can be affected by radiation.

Menopause: If you have not yet experienced menopause, your therapy will induce menopausal changes. You will stop having your period and may develop menopausal symptoms such as hot flashes, insomnia, and mood swings. You should consult your gynecologist to discuss hormonal replacement. Because of changes to the ovaries, you will become infertile and will be unable to have children.

Pati's Comment:

Talk to your doctor if you have not completed your family before you start treatment. It may be possible to save eggs or sperm before radiation. Knowing that radiation can damage ovaries, I had them removed at the time of my colon surgery.

Vaginal Changes: Many women develop vaginal dryness and narrowing in response to radiation therapy. Although this is a permanent problem, it does respond to medical treatment. Using a vaginal moisturizer two to three times a week can decrease dryness, and lubricants can ease soreness during sexual intercourse. It is important, however, to treat the vaginal narrowing that can occur after radiation therapy, either by engaging in sexual intercourse or using a vaginal dilator twice a week. Patients who are not sexually active should still continue to use a vaginal dilator so that necessary vaginal examinations will be possible in the future. Speak to your doctor about how to use a vaginal dilator, and if you are experiencing changes in sexual practice as a result of treatment, you may also want to see a therapist specializing in treating sexual issues (see Questions 89 and 90 for more on coping with sexual changes).

Men

Sexual Dysfunction: Radiation therapy does not cause erectile dysfunction. The risk of erectile dysfunction is related to the extent of surgery necessary to treat rectal cancer, and the potential for damage to nerves leading to the penis. Radiation therapy, however, can cause damage that may limit the amount of sperm and fluid you produce. Patients may notice decreased ejaculate (emission of semen) during intercourse. In addition, sperm counts may be lower, causing infertility. The chance of this happening varies. If you want to conceive children in the future, you should consider using a sperm bank (where you can store your sperm) before radiation therapy and surgery. For more on coping with sexual changes, see Questions 89 and 90.

63. What is brachytherapy?

Brachytherapy

Radiation therapy consisting of the surgical placement of small catheters (hollow tubes) into the body.

With **brachytherapy**, small catheters (hollow tubes) are placed into the body to administer radiation either into or adjacent to where the cancer was situated. This allows the highest therapeutic doses to be given while causing less toxicity to surrounding tissues. It is performed only at specialized institutions that have the necessary resources and equipment available. We limit our use of brachytherapy to patients with locally recurrent colorectal cancer. In many of these patients, external-beam radiation therapy has already been used and has reached the maximum tolerable dose. Brachytherapy allows additional radiation treatments to be given because it causes less toxicity to nearby tissues.

64. What chemotherapy drugs are used for treating colorectal cancer and how are they administered?

We have talked about the role of chemotherapy in question 58. This is an exciting area in the overall management of colorectal cancer because we are seeing rapid improvements every year as scientists understand the mechanisms behind cancer growth. Just within the last five years we have seen the introduction of at least five new agents directed against colon cancer. This is truly amazing progress. With each new discovery we are able to extend the lives of patients with advanced colorectal cancer.

Colon and Colorectal Cancer

The choice of chemotherapy will be based on the location of your cancer (whether colon or rectal), the stage of your cancer, and whether you have other medical conditions. Your surgeon will have you consult a medical oncologist for planning and administration of chemotherapy, and your medical oncologist will work in coordination with your radiation oncologist if radiation treatments are needed. In general, chemotherapy is given as a combination of cytotixic drugs. Combination therapy has consistently proven to be more effective than single drug therapy even in patients with some co-morbid conditions. Combination therapy and a molecularly targeted agents are currently advocated as standard of care for metastatic Stage IV cancers.

Stage III Colon Cancer

Patients with Stage III colon cancer(lymph node involvement) have a high risk for residual cancer cells after surgery. As a result of this high risk of residual cancer after surgery and associated high risk of recurrence, many trials were performed in which advanced chemotherapy effective for more advanced Stage IV cancer were given to patients with Stage III colon cancer after surgery. These trials initially involved chemotherapy with a basic therapy called 5-FU/LV, demonstrating a significant reduction in the risk of recurrent cancer in patients treated with the chemotherapy compared to those who were followed without chemotherapy (approximately a 33% reduction in risk). On this basis, chemotherapy is the recommended post-surgery approach for all Stage III patients.

The current standard of care in treatment of Stage III colon cancer is called FOLFOX* (oxaliplatin-based treatment) based on large clinical trials demonstrating an additional 23% risk reduction of recurrence above and beyond 5-FU/LV alone. Today this therapy is the only FDA-approved combination therapy that has demonstrated efficacy in delaying the progression of the colon cancer in these patients. Since FOLFOX has a proven effect on the cancer in both young and older patients, oncologists prescribe it with confidence to the vast majority of their Stage III patients.

Only in rare instances, when the patient is in very fragile physical condition, a single agent therapy such as 5-FU/LV or capecitabine can be prescribed.

Bolus

A dose of drug given intravenously all at once, rather than by slow infusion.

5-FU is administered intravenously (into a vein) and is either given as a **bolus** (once a week) or as a continuous infusion (by a special pump). For this reason it needs to be administered in the oncologist's office. This type of administration is the most common one for chemotherapies. Bolus infusion is administered more rarely than continuous infusion because studies have shown that bolus infusion can cause more severe side effects. There is also an oral chemotherapy, capecitabine, that the patient can take at home. FOLFOX is administered intravenously on 2 consecutive days every 2 weeks. The infusion can be prolonged for up to 6 hours to ameliorate the potential side effects. Each 2-day administration is called 'a cycle'. The optimal duration of this treatment in Stage III colon cancer is 12 cycles based on large clinical trials.

*Please see important safety information at the end of chapter Treatment. Please see accompanying full prescribing information, including Boxed WARNING.

Table 7 Medications

Name (Trade Name)	Main Use	Side Effects	Comments
5-Fluorouracil (5-FU)	5-FU is the most commonly used drug in the treatment of colorectal cancer. Almost every chemotherapy regimen includes 5-FU. It is used in combination with leucovorin and more recently discovered chemotherapy agents. In Stage III colon cancer, it is combined with oxaliplatin, and in Stage IV colorectal cancer it is combined with oxaliplatin or CPT-11 (irinotecan).	Decreased white blood cell and platelet counts Nausea/vomiting Diarrhea Sores in the mouths and lips Brittle nails Decreased appetite	5-FU, in combination with leucovorin (LV), is the oldest chemotherapy discovered to benefit Stage III colon cancer and Stage IV colorectal cancer patients. It is administered as an intravenous injection.
Leucovorin (Folinic acid; vitamin)	Leucovorin increases the effect of 5-FU. Leucovorin, in combination with both 5-FU, is an established regimen that more recent chemotherapy agents are combined with (see above 5-FU).	Minimal	See above 5-FU. It is administered as an intravenous injection.
Capecitabine (Xeloda)	Xeloda is taken by mouth as a tablet that is broken down inside the body. Xeloda is used as a monotherapy to treat colon cancer after surgery and metastatic colorectal cancer. In studies, Xeloda was no worse than 5-FU/LV but did not improve survival.	Similar to 5-FU Hand and Foot Syndrome Cardiotoxicity Elevated bilirubin levels in blood Contraindicated select patients	Because Xeloda is a tablet and can be taken by mouth, it is viewed as more convenient than injection.
Irinotecan (Camptosar, CPT–11)	CPT-11, alone or in combination with 5-FU/LV, is used to treat cancer of the rectum and colon that has spread to other parts of the body. It is one of the two drugs effective as combination therapies for this stage of cancer.	Decreased blood counts Nausea/vomiting Life-threatening diarrhea Hair loss Abdominal pain Fatigue	CPT-11 is not currently approved in Stage III colon cancer

*Please see important safety information at the end of chapter Treatment. Please see accompanying full prescribing information, including Boxed WARNING.

(continued)

Table 7 continued

Name (Trade Name)	Main Use	Side Effects	Comments
Oxaliplatin* (Eloxitan)	Eloxatin® (oxaliplatin injection), in combination with 5-FU/LV, is indicated for the treatment of Stage III colon cancer. The indication is based on an improvement in disease-free survival, with no demonstrated benefit in overall survival at medium follow up of 4 years. Eloxatin® is also used to treat cancer of the rectum and colon that has spread to other parts of the body.	Nausea, vomiting Numbness and tingling in hands or feet (usually resolves after completion of treatment) Numbness in lips Difficulty swallowing	Oxaliplatin is the only combination chemotherapy approved for Stage III colon cancer.
Mitomycin (Mutamycin)	Mitomycin and 5-FU combined with radiation therapy form the initial therapy for squamous cell carcinoma of the anal canal	Decreased blood counts Nausea, vomiting Poor appetite Fatigue	
Bevacizumab (Avastin)	Avastin is an antibody to Vascular Endothelial Growth Factor (VEG-F). Avastin blocks the formation and growth of new blood vessels feeding the tumor. Avastin is not effective when used alone. It is used in combination with established combination chemotherapy drugs, and has shown to significantly increase their efficacy.	High blood pressure, Kidney problems, Bleeding, Abnormal Blood Clotting	Avastin and Erbitux represent a whole new class known as biologic or targeted events. In recent years they have become an important integral part of treating advanced colorectal cancer in certain patient types. They are not approved by the FDA for the treatment of Stage III colon cancer. They are both still considered experimental and are undergoing further study
Cetuximab (Erbitux)	Erbitux is indicated for the treatment of patients who have colorectal cancer that has spread to other parts of the body. It is used in combination with CPT-11 for patients whose tumor growth progressed after receiving CPT-11. It is also given as a single agent for patients who did not tolerate CPT-11. These patients' tumor expresses a protein called an Epidermal Growth Factor Receptor (EGFR), and Erbitux as an EGFR inhibitor, can be beneficial for them.	Acne like rash, Diarrhea, Allergic Reactions	

*Please see important safety information at the end of chapter Treatment. Please see accompanying full prescribing information, including Boxed WARNING.

Stage IV Colon and Colorectal Cancer

In advanced colorectal cancer, the standard of care in the treatment of advanced Stage IV colorectal cancer is a combination therapy involving chemotherapy and a molecularly targeted drug. There are several combination therapies available which have been determined to be safe and effective. FOLFOX* is the most commonly prescribed combination therapy for these patients. Another combination therapy available is FOLFIRI (a combination of 5-FU/LV and irinotecan).

Recently new drugs have been discovered that are more specific ("targeted") for colon cancer cells. Rather than attacking the cell's nucleus, DNA or RNA and paralyzing its ability to grow, these drugs target other pathways such as circulating growth factors in the body. These factors act as messengers that stimulate a cell to grow. By blocking the factor with a targeted **antibody** the stimulation for cell growth is stopped. Bevacizumab (Avastin) is an antibody directed against circulating vascular endothelial growth factor (VEGF), which works by inhibiting the formation of blood vessels which supply cancer with nutrients and oxygen, and also makes the existing blood vessels supplying the cancer leaky so that chemotherapy delivery can be enhanced. Cetuximab (Erbitux) is an antibody directed against epidermal growth factor receptor (EGFR), which is an important growth factor present in nearly all colon cancers. Both of these are exciting new drugs which have become incorporated in the treatment of patients with metastatic Stage IV colon cancer.

Antibody
Molecule in the body's immune system that identifies foreign substances on bacteria and cancer cells.

Rectal Cancer

Although postoperative chemotherapy and radiation therapy are still used in combination in many centers, the current standard of practice is for preoperative (before surgery) chemoradiation for locally advanced rectal cancer patients.

*Please see important safety information at the end of chapter Treatment. Please see accompanying full prescribing information, including Boxed WARNING.

Treatment includes 5 1/2 weeks of daily radiation therapy with chemotherapy(predominately 5-FU as a continuous IV infusion).

With continuous infusion of 5-FU, a special pump is used that administers chemotherapy continuously over the course of the 5 1/2 weeks in addition to the daily radiation. Continuous-infusion therapy results in less toxicity than bolus regimens, so patients experience fewer or shorter episodes of diarrhea and nausea. Patients therefore tolerate this regimen better and require fewer treatment breaks. With fewer toxic side effects, higher and more consistent doses of chemotherapy can be given, keeping in mind that chemotherapy is a radiation sensitizing agent that helps the radiation work more effectively.

MediPort

Permanent central venous catheter that is placed underneath the skin and usually used for long-term chemotherapy.

Because this kind of chemotherapy is administered 24 hours a day, a more durable intravenous access, called a **MediPort**, is required. A MediPort is placed while the patient is under mild sedation in the operating room or radiology suite. A catheter is placed into one of the large veins in the neck or upper chest and tunneled underneath the chest skin. Because it lies underneath the skin, the risk of infection is less; however, strict sterility is necessary during treatment. A special angled needle is placed into the small reservoir beneath the skin, and chemotherapy can be given through this access. The pump is worn all day and is refilled with medication once a week. Although an invasive procedure is required for placement of the MediPort, continuous 5-FU infusion therapy is becoming increasingly popular because it is less likely to cause toxicity, and because it is more effective than bolus therapy with 5-FU alone.

Stage IV Disease

When a rectal cancer has spread to other organs, like the liver, it is called Stage IV disease. Unfortunately, only rarely does surgery combined with chemotherapy cure Stage IV disease. For this reason, chemotherapy is the first-line treatment instead of surgery, with the hope that a combination of chemotherapy drugs will shrink the tumor and distant deposits so that surgery becomes an option in the future. For Stage IV rectal cancer, treatment is the same as for Stage IV colon cancer.

65. How do I avoid side effects such as infection or diarrhea while receiving chemotherapy?

Compared with chemotherapy for other malignancies, the drugs used for colon cancer treatment are relatively mild and well tolerated. Complete hair loss and severe nausea are uncommon. Many people continue working during treatment with chemotherapy alone. However, even though the toxicity is lower, basic precautions should be taken to prevent unnecessary complications.

Infection: Chemotherapy agents decrease the numbers of circulating white blood cells, which are the body's infection fighters, so you will be more susceptible to common infections. For this reason, you should make efforts to reduce your exposure to infection during chemotherapy. Begin by avoiding people who have symptoms of the flu or other communicable infections. Avoid young children who have recently received live virus vaccinations, including those for polio, measles, and chicken pox. We have some patients who get very preoccupied with "avoiding germs" during their treatments, to the point where they avoid their family members (such as their grandchildren) or stop socializing entirely. However, you should not avoid others altogether, but use common sense in your daily activities. It is important that you enjoy life as much as possible during your treatments, and have social support too, so that you can keep your spirits up.

Make efforts to reduce your exposure to infection during chemotherapy.

Wash your hands frequently, especially before cooking or eating food, and try to maintain strict skin care. You should use skin moisturizers or lotions to prevent dryness and cracking. Attend to cuts and scrapes quickly, and use antiseptics if necessary. Eat well-cooked foods, and avoid undercooked or raw foods like sushi or steak tartare. Make sure eggs are thoroughly cooked, or use frozen, pasteurized eggs for recipes requiring raw eggs. Avoid freshly squeezed juices, unpasteurized beer, and other food items that have not been processed or sterilized (home-grown vegetables, for instance). These simple measures will reduce the risk of stomach upset.

Be on the lookout for symptoms of illness, and seek medical attention quickly. Fever over 100° F (38.2° C) should be reported to your doctor, especially if it is associated with chills and sweats. Redness, heat, and swelling are common signs of a skin infection, especially around an IV site or overlying a MediPort. A sore throat, cough, or very runny nose suggests an upper respiratory infection. Burning on urination can indicate a urinary tract infection and should be treated with oral antibiotics. All of these findings should be reported to your doctor immediately to reduce the risk of further complications.

Pati's Comment:

I was very careful to avoid crowds when my white blood counts were low, but I did need to take antibiotics a few times during chemo. I made sure I drank plenty of fluids to avoid dehydration. I rarely experienced diarrhea but knew to follow the BRAT (bananas, rice, applesauce, toast) diet, keep pushing fluids, and call the doctor if Imodium didn't help control it.

Diarrhea: Diarrhea is the most common side effect of colon cancer chemotherapy. It can be more severe during combined-modality therapy (chemotherapy and radiation). Diarrhea can usually be controlled with variations in diet (Table 8). You should eat smaller but more frequent meals, and choose low-fiber instead of high-fiber foods, which constitutes what is often referred to as a low-residue diet.

Your doctor can prescribe a variety of medications to help with the diarrhea, including Imodium™ or Lomotil™, but initial therapy should focus on modifying your diet. Do not take over-the-counter medication without speaking to your doctor first. Continue to drink plenty of fluids to avoid dehydration. If your diarrhea remains severe, contact your doctor; a liquid diet to give the bowel some rest may be recommended. In severe cases, hospitalization may be required to restore your fluid balance intravenously.

Stomatitis: Stomatitis refers to sores around the mouth and other mucosal surfaces, which are common during treatment with 5-FU. You should see your dentist for an adequate cleaning and examination before you begin therapy. Careful mouth care is the best way to prevent this complication. Brush your teeth regularly, using a toothbrush with soft bristles. Avoid mouthwash that contains salt or alcohol, which may irritate open sores. Choose soft, soothing foods, such as cottage cheese, applesauce, gelatin, ice cream, custards, and scrambled eggs. Avoid spicy, salty, and acidic foods that irritate, like orange or grapefruit juice, lemon juice, and tomatoes, as well as coarse foods, like granola and raw vegetables. In severe cases, topical anesthetics (pain-killers you put directly on the sore area) and -gargles can alleviate difficult symptoms.

Table 8 Dietary recommendations to avoid diarrhea during chemotherapy

Avoid	Choose
Whole grain bread	White bread
Fresh fruits and vegtables	Cooked fruits without the skin
Beans and nuts	White rice
Fiber Cereal	Creamed Cereals
Fried meats	Chicken or turkey without the skin

66. *What about alternative medicine and homeopathic options?*

Approximately half of all cancer patients use alternative therapies.

When diagnosed with cancer, many people turn to unconventional treatments as a last, or even a first, resort in their battle against this disease. However, treatments that were once looked on with skepticism are now enjoying an increase in popularity and acceptance from the public and even the medical community, as long as they are not used to replace conventional treatment. Approximately half of all cancer patients use alternative therapies, and health insurance plans are beginning to cover treatments such as acupuncture. However, some important issues should be considered about these treatments. First of all, they are "complementary" treatments, meaning that they are taken together with current treatments but should never be substituted for conventional medical care. The use of unconventional techniques alone can delay appropriate treatment and can deplete patients' finances before they receive adequate care. That being said, these treatments can improve cancer patients' quality of life by reducing nausea, vomiting, and cancer pain.

Some homeopathic medications contain strong herbal drugs that can interact with conventional medication.

How these treatments work is often poorly understood, and many of the remedies are not under any form of government regulation. Surprisingly, some homeopathic medications contain strong herbal drugs that can interact with conventional medication. If you want to use one of these remedies, you should always consult with your primary physician so that you can be appropriately monitored. An in-depth discussion of complementary medicine is beyond the scope of this book, however, some of the common therapies and their role in cancer management strategies are discussed.

Acupuncture/Accupressure: Acupuncture is the most widely used technique in complementary medicine. By applying needles or external pressure to known pressure points, acupuncturists claim to restore balance in a patient's life force, which can improve health. Studies evaluating acupuncture have had contradictory results. However, good evidence exists that acupuncture helps with the management of back pain, dental pain, migraine, nausea, and vomiting, and in fact, acupuncture may be a beneficial additional treatment for nausea and vomiting caused by chemotherapy. It is a safe procedure, and the complications of infection or pneumothorax (punctured lung) are exceedingly rare.

Herbal Products: Herbal treatments are over-the-counter remedies that contain collections of natural drugs. Although conventional medications usually contain one very pure drug (although they might contain one or more "inert" ingredients that have no effects on the body), herbal therapy often combines a varied cocktail of active drugs. Some herbal products have been tried as chemotherapy agents against cancer. Essiac, a common herbal therapy in North America, contains a combination of burdock, turkey rhubarb, sorrel, and slippery elm. Essiac has not been proven to have an anticancer effect. Iscador, a derivative of mistletoe, has widespread use in Europe. In laboratory studies, mistletoe extracts have shown cancer-fighting properties, although this benefit has not been proved in humans. The only chemotherapy agents proven to have a limited effect against colorectal cancer are the medications that were described earlier in Question 64.

Complementary herbal products, however, can have an adjunctive role in cancer treatment. St. John's wort (Hypericum perforatum) has proven effects in the management of mild depression. Ginger compounds (Zingiber officinalis) may reduce nausea and vomiting. Valerian (Valeriana officinalis) helps some people with insomnia, and kava kava (Piper methysticum) may decrease anxiety. All of these supplements may be bene-ficial in treating the complications of cancer treatments. However, the **Food and Drug Administration (FDA)** does not regulate herbal remedies for safety and effectiveness. In addition, exact drug concentrations may vary widely, and recent reports have revealed significant liver and renal toxicity with some herbal treatments, such as kava kava. Also, the interactions of herbal medications with commercial

Food and Drug Administration (FDA)

The government agency responsible for the approval of medications and new therapies in the United States.

drugs are untested and therefore often unknown. For this reason, herbal medications should be discontinued several weeks before any kind of surgery to prevent unforeseen complications. Similarly, you should discuss any herbal products you are taking with your oncologist if chemotherapy has been recommended for you. Sometimes people take herbal remedies for such symptoms as depression because they feel less stigma is associated with taking herbal remedies than with asking their doctor for help. Counseling and prescription drugs do effectively treat anxiety, depression, insomnia, and other symptoms. Prescription drugs can be safer, and their effects are better known. Speak to your doctor to find the best solutions for you.

Shark Cartilage: Shark cartilage can limit blood vessel growth in laboratory experiments. This has interesting implications for cancer treatment because new blood vessel growth is an important step in tumor growth, so limiting such growth could be important. However, shark cartilage molecules are too large to be absorbed through the human digestive tract, and studies have not demonstrated any benefit from shark cartilage supplementation for patients with advanced cancer.

Diet: There are many advocates for alternative diets that supposedly limit cancer growth. The macrobiotic diet is based on the belief that cancer is the result of an imbalance of yin and yang. The diet seeks to correct this imbalance with foods high in either yin or yang qualities. In practical terms, the macrobiotic changes are similar to USDA recommendations. It encourages the consumption of high-fiber foods, fruits, and vegetables as well as diet supplementation with beans, seaweeds, and soup. Proteins from meats, cheeses, and other processed foods are replaced with soy proteins. Although these dietary changes may help prevent colorectal cancer, there is no evidence that macrobiotic changes will help patients cure their cancer.

The Gerson treatment, popularized in Mexico, uses a combination of diet and other remedies to remove toxins stored in the liver. Treatments include a high-potassium diet, coffee enemas, and daily consumption of a gallon of fruit juice. One study suggested a possible benefit for patients with melanoma, however, the study had many statistical flaws. The clinic's use of raw calf liver injections was recently suspended after several patients developed severe infections. A randomized trial evaluating a restrictive diet with coffee enemas is underway in New York City, but no evidence currently exists to support these treatments as the primary treatment of colon cancer.

Aromatherapy: Aromatherapy is the application of essential plant oils to the body. Although aromatherapy can help relieve the anxiety associated with cancer, it has not been proven to increase life expectancy. Some patients have found that scents such as lavender help them relax during stressful times, such as before chemo or RT treatments.

Spiritual Healing: Spiritual healing is the channeling of energy from an external source (such as God) or from one individual to another, with the intent of physical or emotional healing. Healing can be conferred through direct contact or over a long distance. Reiki and therapeutic touch are examples of spiritual healing techniques. Spiritual healing has not been proven to increase life expectancy in cancer patients. However, two studies have shown that patients who received therapeutic touch had less anxiety and better mental well-being than those who used simple rest periods.

Hypnotherapy: Hypnotherapy can decrease nausea and vomiting in cancer patients and may also reduce cancer pain.

Most physicians welcome complementary treatments when they accompany surgery or other prescribed treatments. You should always tell your doctor if you are using or considering any complementary methods of treating your cancer or related symptoms. Not only will you then be sure that the treatment is safe, but your doctor will also be able to better manage your care.

Kate's Comment:

As soon as people heard that I had cancer, they began to tell me about some natural herb or supplement or special diet that has cured lots of people. "The doctors won't tell you about it," they said, "because there is no profit in something that is natural and cheap." Only these supplements are rarely cheap, and there is no evidence that they work.

After watching friends spend both money and hope on cases of tea, macrobiotic diets that left them hungry and cranky, and even some desperate trips to clinics in Mexico, I began to research every friendly recommendation. A book published by the American Cancer Society, The ACS Guide to Complementary and Alternative Cancer Methods, helped me a lot. I find that some of these alternatives are downright dangerous, some interfere with chemotherapy and healing, and others are just a waste of money. I'd rather spend my money on a good movie or a trip to the beach with my family, simple pleasures that lift my spirits and help me enjoy life.

67. What kind of follow-up will I need after surgery?

Surgery and adjuvant therapy are the primary steps in your battle against colorectal cancer. It is important to try to keep an open mind and a positive attitude because most people's cancer is cured with these therapies. However, you will need to remain vigilant and have good follow-up with your management team, including your primary care physician, gastroenterologist, medical oncologist, and surgeon. The reason for this is twofold. Initial follow-up will be aimed at identifying cancer recurrence. This is done with blood tests and endoscopy, and if after 5 years, you continue to have a clean bill of health, you will be considered "cured" from your primary cancer. However, once you are diagnosed with colorectal can-

If after 5 years, you continue to have a clean bill of health, you will be considered "cured" from your primary cancer.

cer, you are at a higher risk of developing another colorectal cancer later in life. The second goal of follow-up, therefore, is to identify repeat cancers early. You will require frequent colonoscopic screening according to set pro-tocols.

Follow-up is most intensive during the first 3 years after surgery because most recurrences (80%) happen during this time. We recommend seeing a medical specialist, either your surgeon or your on-col-ogist, every 3 months for the first 2 years. At these visits, routine blood tests will be performed to check blood counts and carcinoembryonic antigen (CEA) level. Physical examination will be performed, as well as outpatient procedures such as proctoscopy or sigmoidoscopy, if necessary. These guidelines are flexible. If you ever sense that something has changed, or you simply do not feel well, you should definitely schedule a doctor's appointment sooner. If you are having chronic fatigue, abdominal pain, or abdominal distention, you should seek attention immediately. Changes in your bowel habits still warrant additional workup with colonoscopy. After 3 years have passed from the time of surgery, the interval between follow-up visits can be lengthened to 6 months and then annually after 5 years.

In general, routine surveillance with CT scanning or PET scanning after surgery is not recommended. These tests are expensive, slightly invasive, and have not been proven to help long-term survival. However, patients whose cancers have a high risk of recurrence may undergo follow-up CT scans up to every 6 months for the first 3 years.

Routine follow-up with frequent CEA level testing is recommended. Although clear survival advantages have not been proven with this kind of follow-up, we do know that an elevation in the CEA level occurs in 65% to 75% of all colorectal cancer recurrences. This rise in the CEA level can occur as early as 5 months before physical examination and radiologic tests (x-ray, CT) detect the cancer. Additional testing with CT, MRI, and PET scanning can then be initiated if increases in CEA levels are detected. In a small number of patients, the earlier diagnosis of recurrence by CEA testing may allow a treatment to be used that can improve life expectancy; unfortunately, this is usually the exception rather than the rule. When a cancer recurs, it is often extensive and cannot be cured by conventional methods.

Colonoscopy should be repeated 1 year after surgery so that the surgeon can evaluate the surgical area and check the colon for any new polyps or cancers. If polyps are found, you should have a repeat colonoscopy every 1 to 2 years until the colon is clear. Colonoscopy should then be performed every 3 years.

We advocate an intensive follow-up approach with patients who have tumors of the rectum because they have a higher rate of local recurrence (recurrence in the same area) and also because the site of local recurrence is more accessible for evaluation. After proctectomy, the surgical areas are low down in the rectum and are easily seen by proctoscopy or sigmoidoscopy. Both of these can be performed during routine office visits. We also rely heavily on endorectal ultrasound for patients who have undergone transanal excision of a rectal -cancer. We perform these examinations at every office visit for the first 5 years. Although this is not commonly performed at other institutions, endorectal ultrasound can be a valuable resource in identifying enlarged lymph nodes around the rectum, and it also permits biopsy of suspicious lesions. We recommend routine ultrasound during follow-up visits after transanal excision of rectal cancers (the sphincter-saving surgery in which tumors are removed through the anus).

Pati's Comment:

Your doctors will tell you how often you need to see them. Four years after diagnosis, I now see my GI and radiology oncologist once a year, my oncologist every 6 months. I have had annual CT scans, chest x-rays; CEA, CBC, and metabolic profile every 6 months. My colonoscopy was clear 1 year after diagnosis, so I had a 3-year colonoscopy, which also was clear.

68. What is a PET scan?

Positron emission tomography (PET) is a radiologic examination used to detect recurrent (returning) or metastatic (spreading) cancer. It involves a sugar combined with a small piece of radiation called "FDG-Glucose" which is injected by IV into patients, with the premise that cancer cells are more metabolically active than normal cells, and hence more likely to take up the FDG-Glucose which can be identified by this test. A PET scan can often detect the presence of cancer before CT or MRI.

PET is very accurate in detecting the recurrence (return) of cancer. It can accurately detect liver metastases more than 90% of the time, which is better than CT scanning. Additionally, PET can often distinguish between normal scarring after surgery and actual cancer recurrence, which can be difficult to detect from CT and MRI. Although excellent at identifying recurrence, PET can only be used as an adjunct to CT and MRI, which are needed to create the detailed anatomical images used for planning surgery. Additionally, all abnormal findings on PET scanning need to be confirmed by biopsy and microscopic review.

If you are scheduled for a PET scan, you will need to fast (not eat) the morning of your study; if you eat, the bowel will show elevated levels of activity, which can hide the finding of recurrent cancer. A radioactive substance will be injected into your vein before the PET scanning. The entire study lasts over an hour so that complete recordings can be collected. The image that the PET scan obtains shows "hot spots" that might indicate that the cancer has spread.

PET scanning is a technology still in its infancy. Currently, it is used mainly to help interpret difficult readings on CT and MRI. Newer machines actually combine CT and PET technology for the best of both worlds. Additionally, patients being evaluated for possible surgery if their cancer has recurred have PET studies. If widespread cancer is detected, surgery would be deferred in favor of non-surgical palliative treatment. PET scan is not recommended for routine follow-up or for workup at your initial visit to your doctor.

TREATMENT OF ADVANCED DISEASE

69. What do I do if the cancer has spread to my liver?

The recent improvements in colorectal cancer survival are mostly related to increased screening and earlier diagnosis. Unfortunately, progress has not been as rewarding in the management of Stage IV cancer that has spread to other organs. As many as half of patients who undergo surgery for colorectal cancer will have a return of their cancer, and in these instances, the long-term outlook remains poor. Because the normal blood supply of the colon drains into the liver, most cancer spread (80%) occurs here. Untreated colorectal cancer that has spread to the liver is always fatal, and the average life expectancy is only 5 to 10 months. By the time a tumor has spread to the liver, systemic (whole body) disease is usually present, which cannot typically be treated by surgery; although the entire gross (visible to the naked eye) tumor may be removed, it is likely that small microscopic deposits still remain and can grow at a later time. With this having been said, there is a small group of patients whose metastases in the liver are the only evidence of recurrent tumor. In about one third of these patients, surgical resection of liver metastases can lead to a cure. So although other techniques are available and can improve the patient's quality of live and prolong life expectancy, surgery, when possible, is the only real chance for cure and should be considered when possible.

Only 20% to 30% of patients with liver metastases are candidates for surgery because the cancer has usually spread to other organs as well. In these cases, the disease is truly systemic (throughout the whole body) and cannot be removed surgically. Colorectal cancer also tends to spread to the deep lymph nodes in the abdomen, the lining of the abdominal wall, and the lungs. PET scanning has become a useful study for identifying all sites of disease and determining the appropriateness of the tumor for surgery. When there is spread to other organs, liver surgery is usually not feasible, and systemic chemotherapy (chemotherapy given intravenously and dispersed throughout the body) becomes the treatment of choice.

If your doctor has determined that the tumor is present only in the liver, the next step is to decide whether the tumor can be surgically removed. A surgeon specializing in **hepatic** (liver) surgery will make this decision. The liver is divided into a left and right lobe based on its blood supply, and these lobes are further divided into eight segments. Current surgical techniques allow surgeons to remove small wedges of liver, individual segments, or entire lobes during cancer surgery. Luckily, the liver has the remarkable ability to regenerate, so only 20% of normal liver tissue is needed to function adequately after surgery. The ability to surgically remove liver metastases depends on the size and the location of the tumor inside the liver and its relationship to nearby structures, such as major blood vessels, and CT and MRI scanning of the liver are extremely useful in determining this. Removal of some or part of the liver has become a safe procedure, and the mortality from this procedure is now less than 5% in large treatment centers.

Hepatic
Relating to the liver.

When death occurs, it commonly results from liver failure, if recurrent disease has returned to the liver. A five-criteria system can predict the likelihood that cancer will recur in the liver:

1. The tumor size is greater than 5 cm.
2. The time to spread of cancer to the liver metastases is less than 12 months after primary (first) colorectal surgery.
3. The number of liver tumors is greater than one.

4. The primary (first) tumor has spread to nearby lymph node(s).
5. The preoperative CEA level is greater than 200.

In patients with more than two of these criteria, the cancer in their liver is likely to return. For this reason, these patients may be best treated by primary chemotherapy instead of surgery.

70. Are there other treatments for liver metastases if surgery is not an option?

As we suggested in previous questions, the best possibility for cure in patients with Stage IV colorectal cancer is surgery. However, if surgery is not feasible, the tumor will continue to grow within the liver, causing organ failure and eventually, death. In these cases, other interventions that may increase life expectancy and improve the patient's quality of life may be possible. In the past, systemic chemotherapy (chemotherapy that affects the entire body) has been the mainstay of treatment, and it is the primary therapy for inoperable disease. Combination chemotherapies have recently shown a marked improvement in shrinking the size of the lesions in the liver, and making liver metastases easier to remove with surgery. To achieve that, these combination chemotherapies are given in a limited quantity prior to the surgery, and continued after it.

Hepatic Arterial Infusion Chemotherapy

Hepatic artery infusion (HAI) uses a pump to administer high doses of chemotherapy directly into the blood supply of the liver. In this way, chemotherapy agents can be infused directly into the liver and not dispersed throughout the body with the hope that it would induce a better response than systemic treatments. The liver has two sources of blood: the hepatic artery and the portal vein. Normal liver cells derive most of their blood supply from the portal blood vessels, whereas cancer cells in the liver derive 85-90% of their blood supply from the hepatic arteries. During surgery, a special catheter is placed into the hepatic artery and connected to a chemotherapy pump that is placed underneath the skin. Chemotherapy can be inserted into the pump, and a constant infusion of high doses of chemotherapy is administered directly into the liver.

The reason HAI can be effective is because the liver is the organ that is normally responsible for metabolizing chemotherapy agents. Chemotherapy given intravenously in the arm is spread throughout the body, allowing absorption by all other tissues. Toxicities from these drugs can then occur in other areas, such as the intestines, bone marrow, and oral mucosa (the lining of the mouth). However, the chemotherapy drugs such as floxuridine, given directly into the hepatic artery, have a high "first-pass metabolism". This means that the liver then metabolizes most of the chemotherapy drug (floxuridine) so that very little reaches the blood supply outside the liver. For this reason, much higher doses of total chemotherapy can be administered in this way, and the therapy is focused directly on the tumor cells involved. Fluorodeoxyuridine (FUDR®) is a drug that acts similarly to 5-FU. When given through HAI, over 95% of FUDR® remains in the liver, meaning that less than 5% is dispersed to the rest of the body. Patients receiving HAI have significantly less systemic (body-wide) toxicity, if any at all. Common side effects of systemic chemo-therapy, like diarrhea and stomatitis (irritation of the stoma), are exceedingly rare with HAI.

Tumors are significantly reduced in up to 60% of patients who receive hepatic artery infusion, which is about two times the response of patients receiving only intravenous chemotherapy. In addition, the patient's quality of life is better because fewer side effects occur with HAI. However, HAI is not for everyone. A substantial abdominal operation is required to place the pump. In addition, complications do occur with pump therapy and include bleeding during surgical placement, delayed clotting of the hepatic artery, bile duct scarring (**bilary sclerosis**) and hepatitis.

Bilary sclerosis
Bile duct scarring.

Unfortunately, even HAI will not cure Stage IV colorectal cancer. The tumor can eventually spread beyond the liver and therefore is not affected by the chemotherapy given through the pump. Most protocols, therefore, include systemic chemotherapy given with HAI therapy. In summary, HAI is a useful treatment for colorectal cancer whose spread is limited to the liver and is inoperable by current surgical techniques. HAI can also be used after liver resection to reduce the risk that the cancer will return. Patients with metastases in the liver and elsewhere are candidates for systemic multidrug chemotherapy only.

Judi's Comment:

When my husband was diagnosed with Stage IV colo-rectal cancer that had begun in the rectosigmoid area and spread to the liver, his surgeon implanted an HAI device. Following surgery, my husband received systemic chemotherapy along with HAI directly to the liver. When he was receiving chemotherapy only by way of HAI, his quality of life was very good. He had no side effects during these times and was able to work and enjoy outings with family and friends. According to the literature, HAI buys time, not only extending length but also quality of life. With most Stage IV cancers, metastases finally take over. We knew the odds were not good, but because we also knew of one or two long-term Stage IV survivors, we never lost hope. My husband died nearly 3 years after his surgery, but given his prognosis of living "about a year," I credit HAI with prolonging our time together.

Cryoablation

Cryoablation

An invasive technique that destroys tumor cells through the freezing and thawing of malignant tissue.

Cryoablation is a technique that destroys tumor cells through the freezing and thawing of malignant tissue. Special cryoprobes cooled by liquid nitrogen are inserted directly into the tumor within the liver. Probes as thin as 3 millimeters can freeze a zone of tissue 5 or 6 centimeters in diameter. Most often, cryotherapy is performed during abdominal surgery so the probes can be placed under the surgeon's direct vision into the tumor. However, with the use of newer techniques, cryoprobes can be placed during laparoscopic surgery and even through the skin without a large incision. Although cryoablation is considered less invasive than removal of all or part of the liver, cryotherapy can be complicated by bleeding, liver abscesses, kidney failure, and trauma to other organs.

Aggressive cryotherapy techniques can have mortality of 4%, which is equivalent to that of liver cancer surgery. It should not be considered a harmless procedure, although cryotherapy has been used for many years in the treatment of a variety of liver tumors. It is very effective for killing tumor cells within the freezing zone.

Unfortunately, cryotherapy's usefulness is limited because of the damage it does to adjacent organs and blood vessels. In addition, the reduction in the tumor size by cryotherapy is only temporary, and many tumors return within 6 months. However, cryotherapy remains a useful tool for treating scattered small liver metastases that cannot be removed by surgery. Ongoing trials are currently evaluating the use of cryotherapy in combination with HAI. Currently, liver resection remains the standard therapy for colorectal metastases to the liver, but cryosurgery is a reasonable alternative in selected patients with unresectable disease.

Radiofrequency Ablation

Radiofrequency (RF) ablation uses heat to kill tumors. Like cryoablation, a probe is inserted into the liver and the tumor and an area of surrounding tissue is destroyed with thermal energy. RF is performed with open surgery, laparoscopic surgery, and percutaneous (through the skin) techniques, however, RF and cryotherapy have certain differences. RF is effective in killing tissue only within a 3-cm radius of the probe. Although ultrasound can easily detect the "ice ball" created during cryotherapy, the zone treated by RF is not as easily identified during surgery. Local recurrence is higher.

Radiofrequency (RF) ablation

Cancer treatment that uses heat to kill tumors.

Although the equipment needed to perform RF is much less expensive than that needed for cryotherapy, the role of RF ablation remains to be determined and will depend on technological advances as well as clinical trials with adequate follow-up.

In summary, a variety of established and experimental therapies are available for the treatment of colorectal cancer that has spread only to the liver. These treatments can both lengthen life expectancy and improve the quality of life. Surgical resection, when possible, remains the best opportunity for cure.

71. What is intraperitoneal therapy?

Like HAI, intraperitoneal (inside the abdominal cavity) therapy tries to administer the chemotherapy directly to the tumor deposits. The small bowel and large intestine float freely in a fluid within the abdominal cavity. Although the most common sites for metastatic colorectal deposits include the lymph nodes around the colon, the liver, and the lungs, certain colorectal cancers tend to spread inside the abdomen, covering the lining of the abdominal wall and coating the small and large bowel. This is called carcinomatosis.

Peritoneal cavity
Abdominal cavity.

When the cancer is spread widely within the **peritoneal cavity**, complete removal by surgery is not possible because entire segments of bowel are coated with tumor deposits, and it is impossible to completely remove all tumor deposits and leave enough functional bowel behind. If the bulk of the tumor can be removed by surgery, then administering chemotherapy directly into the abdominal cavity would cause the remaining cancer deposits to be exposed to higher levels of chemotherapy. To administer the treatment, a catheter is placed into the abdomen with a small operation, and chemotherapy agents are injected directly into the abdominal cavity. This is a fairly harmless procedure, however, side effects, including abdominal pain, can occur.

Physicians' experience with intraperitoneal therapy is very limited. There have been a few reports of long-term survivors after intraperitoneal therapy, but few trials have been able to show that this technique improves life expectancy. Intraperitoneal therapy remains an experimental option for a very select group of patients with tumor spread solely to the abdominal cavity.

72. What are the latest developments in the treatment of colorectal cancer?

The struggle against colorectal cancer involves a multisystem approach, including prevention, surgery, and adjuvant treatment techniques. Research is ongoing in all modes of treatment, and many of these have been summarized in previous sections. For example, screening recommendations for colorectal cancer have recently changed, with the trend being toward colonoscopy instead of flexible sigmoidoscopy. Additionally, the introduction of newer techniques, like virtual colonoscopy, may offer less invasive options in the future. Surgical technique has evolved, with the use of total mesorectal excision for rectal cancer, the colonic J-pouch, and sphincter-saving techniques. Genetic testing for hereditary colorectal cancer may allow earlier identification of people who are at risk for the disease, and such testing may help guide management in the future. With a better understanding of the molecular basis of colorectal cancer, new avenues for adjuvant therapy (mainly chemotherapy) are being studied.

The struggle against colorectal cancer involves a multisystem approach.

Oxaliplatin and CPT–11: Oxaliplatin* and CPT–11 have recently been incorporated in the treatments for colorectal cancer, and patients taking these drugs have had excellent responses after not responding to treatment with 5-FU. Oxaliplatin or irinotecan in combination with 5-FU and leucovorin are now standard treatments for Stage IV colorectal cancer patients, sometimes given with newer molecularly targeted drugs such as bevacizumab.

*Please see important safety information at the end of chapter Treatment. Please see accompanying full prescribing information, including Boxed WARNING.

5-FU/LV: 5-FU/LV is a mainstay of chemotherapy for both Stage III colon cancer and advanced colorectal cancer patients. In Stage III colon cancer 5-FU/LV is used in combination with oxaliplatin*, and in advanced colorectal cancer 5-FU/LV is used in combination with either oxaliplatin or CPT-11. The use of 5-FU/LV alone is appropriate only in very elderly and fragile patients. 5-FU is given by continuous infusion because this method is effective, has low toxicity, and allows high doses to be given; however, this treatment requires that a permanent access port be placed because a pump is used. An oral form of 5-FU, capecitabine, has been approved as a substitute for intravenous techniques, with recent studies demonstrating non-inferiority.

Molecularly Targeted Therapy: More recently, new targeted therapeutic agents have jumped into the limelight and have become incorporated in the standard treatment of patients with Stage IV colon and rectal cancer.

However, newer techniques use antibodies against growth factors in the body that are needed by all cells for growth. For example vascular endothelial growth factor (VEGF) is a chemical in the body that stimulates the growth of blood vessels. Because cancer cells grow so quickly, they need more nutrients and so induce blood vessels to grow into the tumor. By blocking VEGF with a targeted antibody the stimulation for blood vessel growth is stopped and the tumor cannot receive enough nutrients. Bevacizumab (Avastin) is an antibody directed against the circulating vascular endothelial growth factor (VEGF) which has been FDA approved for use in combination with chemotherapy for patients with Stage IV colon or rectal cancer. Cetuximab (Erbitux) is an antibody directed against epidermal growth factor receptor (EGFR), an important growth factor responsible for the growth and spread of colon and rectal cancers, which has also been FDA approved for use in a specific group of Stage IV colon and rectal cancer patients who have irinotecan resistant disease. Both of these exciting new drugs are available for Stage IV

*Please see important safety information at the end of chapter Treatment. Please see accompanying full prescribing information, including Boxed WARNING.

colorectal cancer and are under evaluation in combination with many newer drugs.

The treatment of colorectal cancer is constantly changing. Newer technologies for screening, surgical techniques, and adjuvant techniques have led to better life expectancy in people with colorectal cancer. If you are diagnosed with advanced cancer, ask your oncologist about ongoing trials and whether you need to be referred to a larger, specialized cancer center.

Important Safety Information

What is ELOXATIN® (oxaliplatin injection)?
ELOXATIN (eh-LOX-ah-tin) is an anticancer (chemotherapy) medicine that is used with other anti-cancer medicines called 5-fluorouracil (5-FU) and leucovorin (LV):

- to treat adults with stage III colon cancer after surgery to remove the tumor,
- to treat adults with advanced colon or rectal cancer (colorectal cancer).

ELOXATIN with infusional 5-FU and LV was shown to lower the chance of colon cancer returning when given to patients with stage III colon cancer after surgery to remove the tumor. It is not known if ELOXATIN increases survival in patients with stage III colon cancer. ELOXATIN with infusional 5-FU and LV was also shown to increase survival, shrink tumors and delay growth of tumors in some patients with advanced colorectal cancer.

The use of ELOXATIN in children has not been studied.

Who should not use ELOXATIN?
Do not use ELOXATIN if:

- You are allergic to platinum. The active ingredient in ELOXATIN is oxaliplatin, which is a platinum-containing drug. Cisplatin (Platinol®) and carboplatin (Paraplatin®) are other chemotherapy medicines that also contain platinum.
- You are pregnant. ELOXATIN may harm your unborn child. You should avoid becoming pregnant while taking ELOXATIN. Talk with your doctor about how to avoid pregnancy.

Tell your doctor if you are breast feeding. We do not know if ELOXATIN can pass through your milk and if it can harm your baby. You will need to decide whether to stop breast feeding or not to take ELOXATIN. Tell your doctor about all the medicines you take, including prescription and non-prescription medicines and herbal supplements. ELOXATIN may affect how they work in your body.

What are the possible side effects of ELOXATIN?

ELOXATIN can cause allergic reactions.
Get emergency help right away if: You suddenly have trouble breathing. Your throat feels like it is closing up.
Call your doctor right away if you have any of the following: Other signs of allergic reaction; rash, hives, swelling of your lips or tongue, sudden cough
Call your doctor if you get any of the following: Fever or signs of infection (redness and swelling at the intravenous site, pain on swallowing, cough that brings up mucous, sore throat, shivering, pain on urination), vomiting that is

persistent, diarrhea (frequent, loose, watery bowel movements), signs of dehydration (too much water loss), tiredness, thirst, dry mouth, lightheadedness (dizziness), decreased urination

Tell your doctor if you get a dry cough and have trouble breathing (shortness of breath) before your next treatment. These may be signs of a serious lung disease.

ELOXATIN can affect how your nerves work and make you feel (peripheral neuropathy). Tell your doctor right away, if you get any signs of nerve problems listed below: Very sensitive to cold temperatures and cold objects, trouble breathing, swallowing, or saying words, jaw tightness, odd feelings in your tongue, or chest pressure, pain, tingling, burning, (pins and needles, numb feeling) in your hands, feet, or around your mouth or throat, which may cause problems walking or performing activities of daily living. The first signs of nerve problems may occur with the initial treatment. The nerve problems can also start up to 2 days afterwards. If you develop nerve problems, the amount of ELOXATIN in your next treatment may be changed. Other common side effects from ELOXATIN include nausea, vomiting, diarrhea, constipation, mouth sores, stomach pain, fever, loss of appetite, and tiredness.

These are not all the possible side effects of ELOXATIN. For more information, ask your doctor or pharmacist. Paraplatin® and Platinol® are registered trademarks of Bristol-Myers Squibb Company.

PART FIVE

Changes Cancer Makes

Why is it important to learn how to effectively cope with my diagnosis of colorectal cancer?

How do I know whether I am making the best treatment decisions regarding my newly diagnosed colorectal cancer?

Between my appointments, I think of many important questions to ask my doctor, but when I finally get into the exam room, I get intimidated and distracted. How can I be more relaxed and better express myself to the medical team?

More . . .

MAKING IMPORTANT DECISIONS

73. Why is it important to learn how to effectively cope with my diagnosis of colorectal cancer?

Cancer. Colorectal. Surgery. Chemotherapy. Radiation. When you hear these words, your mind is initially filled with many images, thoughts, and feelings—all of which affect your ability to cope with a diagnosis of colorectal cancer. After learning about the medical aspects of the disease from your doctor and other sources, such as the earlier questions addressed in this book, you may feel stunned and overwhelmed. However, with information and guidance, you can modify negative thoughts and feelings, and, we hope, move forward with confidence in your ability to deal with your diagnosis of colorectal cancer.

Living with cancer includes learning how to cope.

Living with cancer includes learning how to cope with the practical and emotional aspects of your diagnosis, as well as learning how to treat your cancer with surgery and/or other medical treatments. The emotional impact of cancer may be overlooked by medical staff and subsequently by patients themselves and their families. Developing coping skills is a challenging learning process—but when you cope more effectively, reduce anxiety, and focus on enhancing your quality of life, you will manage your medical care effectively and also feel better. The issues you may face as you begin to cope with colorectal cancer may include:

- Orientation to your medical team
- Communication with your medical team, family, and friends
- Common emotions and reactions
- Ways to help reduce distress and increase quality of life
- Family and caregiver concerns
- Home care
- Financial, insurance, and employment issues
- Community resources

If you do not find all of the information in this section helpful now, you may in the future. After discussing various methods of alleviating distress with your doctor and your loved ones, keep an open mind about what might help you feel better and lead a better quality of life. You are facing something completely new so it also may be necessary to remain open to new ideas and ways to help.

74. How do I know whether I am making the best treatment decisions regarding my newly diagnosed colorectal cancer?

After the initial diagnosis, you will have to make medical decisions while under a lot of stress and sometimes uncertainty about what the "right" decisions are. Learning how to manage your medical care is a crucial step toward effective decision making. As you are making important decisions, your stress levels are higher, and you are absorbing a huge amount of information about cancer. If you have just been diagnosed with cancer, you may consider seeking a second opinion from a cancer specialist in your area, ideally from a colorectal surgeon who routinely performs cancer surgery. Don't hesitate to seek a second opinion. Your doctor should not object to this decision; in fact, your doctor should support it. However, do try to refrain from seeking too many "second opinions" because this can delay treatment and add to your confusion regarding the best course of treatment.

Don't hesitate to seek a second opinion.

Choose the right doctor for you. Many factors will influence your decision, including the physician's experience treating colorectal cancer and his or her technical skills, the hospital's location, your insurance coverage, and personal factors, such as the physician's ability to gain your trust and confidence (or "bedside manner"). Interview prospective surgeons and other physicians; assess their experience and other criteria that you consider important.

Identify how much you personally want to know about your cancer, such as stage of disease, progression, and so on. If you are the type of person who would rather not know the details, designate one or two family member(s) to attend appointments with you to gather necessary information and serve as a "point person" through whom the medical team can communicate openly.

Discuss external information sources directly with your doctor who is a partner in your care. Topics of discussion for your doctor may include personal research from books or the Internet. Do not solely rely on chat rooms, personal testimonials, or the thousands of cancer resources that exist because many of them are unreliable (see our Appendix on page XX containing reliable, useful resources). Even on reliable Web sites, statistics and medical information can be confusing and shocking. Filter all information through your doctor to get the real story, to clarify concerns, and to get the answers to your questions regarding your treatment.

You may be presented with several options regarding treatment, and the medical team may leave the final decision up to you. Some people like being able to make this decision; they feel that they are actively involved in their care. Others, however, are confused and anxious about making such important medical decisions. First, clarify the pros and cons with the medical team, including the factors that affect your quality of life. For example, does one chemotherapy regimen have more side effects than the other, even though both may be equally effective in treating the cancer? You may consider discussing the options with people close to you. Clarifying the issues, having support, and sharing the burden of decision making can take pressure off you. Remember that you have the final say and that you are the one who will have to live with whatever decisions you make. You may never know the one "right" decision to make, as is common with many decisions in life. Don't put too much pressure on yourself. Make an informed decision with the assistance of the medical team and then move forward.

Tip: Use the questions presented in this book as a guide to what questions to ask your doctor.

75. Between my appointments, I think of many important questions to ask my doctor, but when I finally get into the exam room, I get intimidated and distracted. How can I be more relaxed and better express myself to the medical team?

Pati's Comment:

The best advice is to jot things down as you think of them. I used to hand my doctor a copy of my list of questions and we would go through the list one by one. My blood pressure was always higher than normal at these appointments, too. I tried to relax with deep breathing.

The interaction between you and your medical team is a crucial aspect of your care and can be most helpful to you when you are dealing with these important treatment decisions. If you are feeling vulnerable, there are several things you can do to make yourself more comfortable.

- Identify what you think and how you feel about your doctor. Is he or she intimidating or likable? Does your doctor use complex terms that you don't understand? Are you afraid of what he or she will find or say about your cancer? Answers to such questions can point you in the right direction for overcoming any negative feelings you may have. Discuss concerns you have directly with your physician; many problems can be solved, which can help you feel more comfortable. If your feelings are interfering with your ability to get appropriate medical care, you may consider finding another physician to treat you.

- Write your questions down before you come to the appointment, in order of most important to least important. You may also want to record by date any physical observations you have made about yourself since your last visit, such as possible side effects of your treatment or medications, including pain, fatigue, nausea, sleeplessness, and/or any other body changes. Also tell your doctor if you are feeling sad, depressed, or anxious.
- Document your doctor's answers and instructions, or use a tape recorder so that you will remember important points after you leave the exam room. Be sure to ask your doctor's permission first before using recording devices.
- Ask someone with whom you are comfortable to come with you so that you have another set of ears listening to what the doctor says. This person can serve as support and as your advocate, particularly if you feel sick, have concerns about expressing yourself, or feel overwhelmed by the information.

Be honest with the medical team about your symptoms.

- Be honest with the medical team about your symptoms and about how you are feeling. Some people want to "hide" the side effects of their treatment for many reasons. For example, they may think that the doctor will put them on a lower dose of treatment, which will make it less likely to cure the cancer, or they fear that their cancer is growing if they feel bad. Still other people are concerned about appearing "weak" to the doctor. You need to be able to trust your doctor to treat your cancer; you should also trust your doctor with the truth about how you feel.
- Ask for clarification if you do not understand what your doctor is saying. Oncology physicians are experts in treating cancer, but sometimes they communicate differently than you do. If you do not understand, do not feel embarrassed to ask, ask, and ask again. Nurses

are specially trained to educate you about medical issues and address many routine concerns. Asking the clinical nurse to clarify information in plain terms can be extremely helpful.
- Ethnic and cultural differences may exist between you and your medical team; these differences may make communication difficult and add to any initial mistrust you may feel. If you have questions or concerns about these issues, talk to your hospital social worker or another health care professional with whom you feel comfortable.
- If your primary language is not English and you are being treated in the United States, your stress may be even higher because of difficulty in communication. Try to bring a family member or friend who can interpret for you. Additionally, hospitals should have staff or volunteer translators available for many languages; if they do not, investigate into using an electronic translator or an electronic dictionary, particularly in emergency situations. Phone translation services are also available from some companies, such as LanguageLine Services (see Question 100 for contact information).

Your health care team is composed of different professionals who are specially trained to deal with the medical and emotional issues you are confronting. Become familiar with these people and the ways they can help you. The following is a list of the standard team members and what they can do for you.

- Physicians and surgeons (MDs). May include a medical oncologist (expert in chemotherapy, among other cancer treatments), a surgeon, and/or a radiation oncologist (expert in radiation treatments). There are many additional doctors and specialists who may be involved in your diagnosis of cancer and/or treatment. If you are unfamiliar with the different terms used to describe these specialists, ask for clarification.

- Nurses. Registered nurses (RNs) typically have a 4-year college degree and hospital training. They are an integral part of your care and will be helpful to you. Nurses provide patient care on the inpatient floors and outpatient clinics, and they can be very specialized in the type of care they provide. A nurse practitioner (NP) is an advance practice clinician with a master's degree who can prescribe medications and write medical orders (in most states), provide direct medical care, and serve as a good resource for routine questions; a clinical nurse specialist (CNS) is a nurse with a master's degree who can provide patient care, but also specializes in the role of an educator in a medical specialty. Depending on your state and hospital policies, other people may be involved in different types of hands-on patient care, including licensed practical nurses (LPN), nursing assistants, and patient certified technicians (PCT).
- Physician Assistants (PA). PAs are medical professionals who can diagnose, treat, and write prescriptions and medical orders, all under the supervision of a physician. Many clinics and hospitals employ both PAs and NPs to assist the physicians treating your cancer.
- Social workers (LMSW, LCSW, LSW). In most states, certified or licensed social workers usually have at least a master's degree (MSW, MSSW). They are available to assist you in coping with your diagnosis, the stress of adjustment to treatment and hospitalization, and can provide counseling to you and your family. They may also help you identify community resources and may coordinate your discharge from the hospital.
- Case managers (or discharge planners). Some hospitals have nurse case managers who are responsible for coordinating your discharge from the hospital, whereas at other hospitals social workers perform this role. Find out who performs this role at your hospital so that you

can contact that person to discuss home care, equipment, facility placement (such as a nursing home), or other discharge needs.

- Interns/residents/fellows. If you are being treated at a teaching hospital, you may have a variety of "doctors-in-training." These team members can often be helpful and supportive of you. Remember, however, that the attending physician is the person who is in charge of your care and that if you have questions or think that you have been given inconsistent information you can ask to speak directly to the attending doctor in charge of your care.
- Enterostomal therapy specialist or ostomy nurse specialist. This person is usually a nurse with special training in ostomy care, including coping with body changes after surgery. Ideally, if you plan to have an ostomy, this specialist will meet with you both before and after your surgery to help you participate in caring for your ostomy and to address your questions.
- Clinical dietitians/nutritionists. They are available to provide education on the role of diet in your recovery from cancer. They are often part of the inpatient medical team and sometimes are available in outpatient clinics as well. You may want to contact one of these professionals to answer any questions you may have on what foods to eat, how to prepare food, and what food to avoid during or after your treatments.

Hospitals also employ many other experts who may be involved in your care, such as patient advocates/representatives, physical therapists, respiratory therapists, occupational therapists, psychologists, psychiatrists, other physician specialists, hospital chaplains, technicians, and patient escorts. You may want to get to know the people involved in your care. By making a personal connection, you may feel more comfortable and supported by those around you.

EMOTIONAL STRESSES

76. After being diagnosed with cancer, I have had a variety of emotional reactions. Is this normal or am I going crazy on top of having cancer?

Pati's Comment:

Cancer puts you on a wild roller coaster ride like nothing else. How could you not be affected by cancer?

Every individual's reaction to cancer is just that—individual. People have both negative and positive reactions to adversity, including a diagnosis of cancer. These reactions may include the following:

- Asking yourself why you got cancer
- Feeling more isolated and alone
- Feeling vulnerable and/or less able to control aspects of your life
- Being less able to concentrate
- Blaming yourself for your diagnosis
- Viewing your body and yourself differently
- Experiencing changes in your relationships with family members and friends
- Redefining life priorities
- Reevaluating spiritual beliefs

Common emotions felt by people who have been diagnosed with cancer include fear of the future, of pain, of loss, of death; anger, either diffuse (general) or directed at particular situations or people; guilt, for believing they are responsible for putting their families through their diagnosis, and for "imposing" on others for care and support; and love and gratitude toward people close to them. A cancer diagnosis often brings people closer to their loved ones. Patients often relate that they feel more connected and that they love their family even more than before their diagnosis as a result of reevaluating life's priorities. For many people, priorities change after their diagnosis, allowing them to focus on spending time with their significant others and on their love for one another.

Sometimes fluctuations in mood can result in "blow-ups," such as bickering with loved ones, overreacting to daily hassles (such as traffic, your child spilling something), other times just yelling, feeling very angry, or crying abruptly for "no reason." Many people do not have full insight into how their daily levels of stress, or distress, contribute to such behaviors. Think of stress as cumulative—it has a way of adding up. And this build-up of stress can make people react more strongly to a situation than they would have otherwise. Sometimes, the situations do not seem particularly upsetting on the surface, but they bring out a strong emotional response. For example, Jack, a businessman, age 57, initially met with his hospital social worker to get help reducing his "hidden" stress. He said:

"I thought that I was dealing with my cancer well—I did not let it get me down and I did not ever cry. I went through a lot, though. I had some complications after surgery, and then I found out that I needed chemo. After I started back to work and taking chemo once a week, I started to feel a little more "edgy," is how I describe it; I was even losing sleep. However, I thought that I was still doing OK. That is, until I found myself getting really annoyed at small things. And I knew that I wasn't doing 'OK' when I snapped at my young granddaughter for spilling her juice. This was totally out of character for me. I guess that my feelings were just building up, and they did come out, but not in a good way."

Jack later talked about how he really felt after his diagnosis and through his surgery and chemotherapy. He felt angry at having cancer, overwhelmed by the complications, treatment, and other responsibilities, and he felt guilty for having put his family through his medical problems. He believed that he was the provider and that he was not supposed to be the dependent one. He tried to maintain the stoic image to others so that he could maintain his self-image as a strong man. However, it finally caught up to him, and his "trigger" happened to be his grandchild's accidental spill. If you find yourself releasing emotions in similar ways, you may find stress-reduction techniques helpful as well as other forms of counseling. Jack needed to meet with his social work counselor only a couple of times to gain insight into the role that stress and his feelings played in his life. He learned coping techniques, which helped him gain better control over his reactions to these feelings. He also learned to focus on his love for his family and to use **positive coping** methods (see Questions 77 and 81) to help him focus on the good things in his life that help deflect the negative experiences.

Positive coping

A term the author uses to refer to a person's unique methods of managing distress, including focusing on a positive attitude, in addition to identifying and addressing the negative reactions to having cancer.

77. I have heard that "positive thinking" can help cure my cancer. Is this true?

"Sometimes I don't feel so positive, and the rest of [my] family gets upset with me when I express negative thoughts, such as speculating whether the surgery and treatments actually will work, or sometimes wondering whether it is worth going through all this. Now, I am not only feeling guilty about having negative thoughts because I believe that I may be hurting my chances of survival, but I also feel like I am letting my family down."

—Jean, age 46, high school teacher, diagnosed with colon cancer

One of the most common questions from patients and their family members is about the role of "positive thinking." Sometimes people believe that thinking positively all the time is necessary. They then feel guilty when they cannot perform this impossible task, because they think that they are negatively affecting their cancer or their chances of survival by periodically having a negative attitude. Research has shown that stress and/or other emotional reactions can lead to specific changes in people's hormone levels, can affect certain types of immune functioning, and may influence other medical problems, such as heart disease. However, research has not yet found a conclusive cause-and-effect relationship between positive thinking, personality characteristics, and/or coping styles and cancer development, diagnosis, or prognosis (prediction of the course of your disease). The relationship between mental events and physical events is not clearly understood; thinking negatively or positively has not been proven to directly affect colorectal cancer growth or cure cancer. It is similarly unlikely that you gave yourself cancer by having certain personality characteristics, being depressed, or being stressed.

What we do know is that mood and other emotional factors may lead to behaviors that promote health; these behaviors may, in turn, indirectly enhance life expectancy. For example, if a person is eternally pessimistic and hopeless, he may postpone important medical tests, such as a colonoscopy, or treatment because he erroneously believes that negative outcomes are inevitable. Therefore, delaying medical attention may affect the likelihood that the cancer is treated successfully.

Even though positive thinking may not directly affect your cancer, some people find that maintaining a hopeful, positive outlook does make them feel better. Positive thinking can help decrease distress, which can in turn make a person better able to handle treatments and possible side effects. You can help yourself through difficult times by viewing life as worth living, seeking enjoyment, connecting with others, and seeing yourself as a fighter who will survive. Remember, however, that trying to think positively all the time is simply not possible and can cause undue stress.

Positive coping, not just positive thinking. Expressing a healthy mix of positive and negative thoughts and emotions is normal. Balance your emotions by focusing on the positive but not ignoring the unpleasant thoughts; think of this as "positive coping" not merely "positive thinking." As you become more comfortable with this process, your family may start to feel more comfortable with you expressing a mix of both positive and challenging reactions.

Furthermore, suppressing negative thoughts and emotions often does not work because people tend to think more about the very thing they try to forget. In other words, the more you resist an emotion or thought, the stronger it may become. If you find yourself thinking unpleasant thoughts, first of all, do not judge yourself for thinking them. Second, take a moment to focus on them to help identify what is truly bothering you. Do you picture a certain image, such as an unpleasant medical procedure? A recurring scenario or a particular worry? Sometimes talking about the unpleasant thoughts is a good way of getting to the heart of the issue, and this can help you resolve the problem. Third, if you find yourself frequently thinking and/or talking about a particular worry, you may want to take action to help yourself, either by solving the problem (if possible) or seeking professional help from a mental health professional to help you cope better with the problem.

Do not try to radically change your personality if you consider yourself generally a pessimistic person since this would be impossible. If you are confused about whether you are "thinking properly," need help with positive coping, or would like advice on how to better communicate with your family members, speak to your social worker, pastoral counselor, or other mental health professional for guidance.

78. I feel as though my life is out of control after my diagnosis of colorectal cancer. How can I regain control of my life?

Kate's Comment:

I felt completely out of control when I was first diagnosed with colon cancer. I was in the hospital, in pain, and scared. My husband and children were trying to manage on their own. I had left work unfinished in my office. I had no idea what was happening or what the future held. Little by little, I began to take hold of what I could control. Getting out of bed and walking after surgery helped me do something for my own healing.

Loss of control is a common feeling for cancer patients. Most aspects of your life are going to be disrupted, at least temporarily. You may feel that your own body has turned against you and that body functions that were once automatic may now be less in your control. People with colorectal cancer may have difficulty when bowel movements are altered, appetite or weight fluctuates, pain is not well-managed, and/or their bodies are altered from surgery and other treatments. Attending medical appointments, dealing with insurance, and many other issues disrupt your usual routines, and the side effects of treatment (possibly including nausea, fatigue, weight changes) may alter your ability to socialize or to do other things you used to do.

These disruptions associated with cancer diagnosis leave some people feeling frustrated and depleted. Try to remember that many of these effects are temporary and will subside. Be aware that concerns about control in some areas may sometimes lead people to believe that all things are out of their control. This simply is not true. Help yourself by focusing on what you can control, including engaging in enjoyable activities (either old or new ones), asking for assistance when needed, and learning about ways that you can help yourself (see Questions 81 and 82), including ostomy care, exercise, and diet, if appropriate. Remember that learning more about your disease, its treatment, and the side effects of treatment, and becoming more involved are all important steps toward normalizing your life and taking back control.

Kate's Comment:

Learning to control what I can and let the rest go has been the most important lesson that cancer has taught me. I have little control over whether my cancer will return, although I can keep a close watch on my health so it is found early. I have almost no control over when I die, although I can make decisions about when it will be right to stop active treatment. I have no control over the reactions and fears of other people. I can do much to improve my own life, however, to fill it with balance and beauty, fun and laughter. I can also find meaningful things to do, although illness now leaves me unable to work full- time. Reaching out to other people with cancer, through support groups and online discussion groups, has been a huge help in giving my life meaning and purpose.

Tip: You do have control over how you are going to cope with cancer. When you feel you do not have control, take control by asking for help.

79. Who is at higher risk to experience difficulties in coping with cancer?

Some people go through their entire diagnosis and treatment able to maintain a generally positive outlook, manage their medical care while balancing their daily lives, and cope well with their diagnosis and side effects of treatment. Anyone, however, may experience difficulty coping. The following situations or characteristics may increase people's distress:

- Past negative experiences with medical treatments or hospitals
- Recent or unresolved losses (including deaths, divorce, job loss)
- Loss of family (or friend) to cancer or personal history of previous cancer diagnosis
- Personal or family history of depression, anxiety, or other psychiatric diagnosis
- History of drug or alcohol abuse
- Initial cancer diagnosis at an advanced stage
- Lack of spirituality, religious views, or meaningful life philosophy
- Particularly stressful lifestyle before diagnosis
- Financial concerns

- Generally pessimistic view toward life or feeling overwhelmed when faced with life challenges
- Past or current trauma (war combat or physical or sexual abuse)
- Responsibility for minor children or dependent adults
- Elderly or disabled and living alone; lack of social supports; being isolated

If you identify one or more of these situations and think that they will increase your distress as you cope with your cancer, consider being proactive by seeking advice from a mental health professional or attending a support group. By asking for help in the beginning, you may be able to prevent distress from getting worse by learning how to manage your feelings; this will help you to solve some of the problems interfering with successful coping. Further information about types of support and counseling are discussed in Question 82.

80. How do I know if my distress has reached a level at which I need professional help?

Periodic mood swings and distress are normal after a diagnosis of cancer and during your treatments. However, for some people these normal reactions may become severe enough for a person to experience symptoms of clinical depression, anxiety disorders such as phobias or panic attacks, or other treatable psychological problems. In fact, some researchers estimate that as many as 25% to almost 50% of cancer patients experience clinically significant distress. If you feel "down" for more than several consecutive weeks, or if unsettling moods interfere with your ability to function in daily life, then contact your doctor or social worker to discuss possible ways to help. If you have a history of abusing or misusing drugs or alcohol, and/or a psychiatric diagnosis, or even have had episodes of feeling depressed or anxious that have not been officially diagnosed, you could be particularly susceptible to depression, anxiety, or the misuse of drugs during the stress of this illness.

Review the list of symptoms provided for depression and anxiety disorders (Table 9). This list is not comprehensive, and it is not intended for self-diagnosis; it is intended to educate you about the possible symptoms of depression and anxiety disorders (which can occur simultaneously). There are many other psychological diagnoses that have different symptoms. Sometimes it is hard to distinguish between the physical side effects of certain treatments or symptoms related to the cancer itself and the symptoms of distress. Therefore, if you experience the symptoms listed, or if you have others that are not listed, ask your physician and/or a mental health professional to accurately diagnose and treat you so that you can start to feel better. A description of different types of mental health professionals is provided in Question 82.

Table 9 Symptoms of depression and anxiety

- Sleep disturbances
- Appetite changes, weight fluctuation
- Little enjoyment of activities that you used to like
- Increased thoughts about death, hopelessness, and/or thoughts or plans of suicide
- Feeling fatigued or having little energy
- Being physically slowed down or the opposite, feeling nervous or restless
- Depressed mood or sadness, tearfulness
- Feeling alone and isolating yourself from others
- Being less able to concentrate or make decisions
- Feeling worthless or guilty
- Uncontrollable or excessive anxiety or worry
- Fear or "phobia" of a certain situation or event (needles, blood draws)
- Being more irritable or agitated
- Engaging in compulsive behaviors (e.g., seeking reassurance by repeatedly asking the same questions)
- Feeling muscle tension
- Mentally and emotionally re-experiencing past upsetting events

Derived from Diagnostic and Statistical Manual of Mental Disorders, 4th Edition (DSM-IV).

81. Are there any useful techniques to help me manage the stress of my diagnosis, upcoming surgery, and possible chemotherapy and radiation therapy?

Pati's Comment:

I found strength through my religious practice—meditation and prayer. I listened to music, often wearing my earphones as I waited for treatments. After I left the hospital, I walked outside every day. I found a special walk along an old canal, full of flowers. Walking eased anxiety and gave me energy.

Identify past coping techniques. Start by looking back on how you have coped with difficult situations in the past. People tend to use the same coping methods to deal with difficult, but different, situations. Ask yourself whether your methods of coping have been productive and effective. As long as you did not use negative forms of coping, such as drug or alcohol abuse, overeating or under-eating, or violent behavior, you may find that your past coping strategies may be most effective now: remember that you are the best expert on what you need to cope the best, and in addition to your past coping methods, you may choose to try the following "positive coping" techniques.

Use social support. An important coping method for many people is using the social support of friends, family, colleagues, or others in your "immediate world." If possible, identify one or two people with whom you can openly share your feelings and fears. Sometimes, talking about your thoughts, feelings, and concerns is one of the best ways to get things off your chest, problem solve, and obtain help from others.

Live life. Identify some people as "fun activity partners," meaning people who you can just be with, without necessarily talking about your cancer. Go to the movies, go out to dinner, or play golf with these people. Identify other supports and good distractions in your life, such as attending religious services, going to work, spending time with your family and friends, or taking up a new hobby or class. You can also do small things for yourself, like buying yourself something fun and spontaneous—a gossip magazine, a CD from a completely new artist, or a new electronic gadget. If your appearance is important to you, you can buy a wig (if you are expecting hair loss due to treatments) or new beauty products to make you feel better. Ask yourself what you love in your life and what you enjoy the most. After you identify these things, do them. Now. Live life! You are fighting for your life, so take time to enjoy the very thing you are fighting for.

Live life! You are fighting for your life, so take time to enjoy the very thing you are fighting for.

Live within limits. You may feel frustrated by the new limitations your body places on you while you "live life," such as fatigue or other symptoms during your treatments or after surgery. Pace yourself, and make adjustments according to how you are feeling. This requires a mental adjustment of how much your body can handle now versus what it could handle before cancer treatment. For example, you may enjoy seeing movies, but you may not have enough energy to make a trip to the theater. Rent a movie instead and stay at home. You may have enough energy some nights to watch only part of the movie. This is OK. Your body needs rest to recuperate, and pushing yourself past your limits can be counterproductive, making you more fatigued and stressed.

Focus on the spiritual. Often, people need help answering difficult questions that arise about their spirituality and beliefs—they may sometimes even question long-held beliefs. Many people wonder why they were diagnosed with cancer, and they speculate about whether they are being punished or tested. These thoughts are common, but they can also create added anxiety if left unaddressed. Your faith and the strength you get from your spirituality may be a crucial part of coping with your diagnosis. If you belong to a religious group, or if you attend services, you may also find further support from others in your religious community. Many people with cancer have been comforted by their own prayers and by knowing that others are praying for them to recover. You may choose to meet with a hospital chaplain or use your own spiritual support system to explore meaning in your life and your diagnosis, and to begin to understand your current experiences in the context of your own beliefs. Even if you are not religious or spiritual, you may have philosophical concerns you may want to discuss with a hospital chaplain or someone else you trust.

Keep active. Under the supervision of your doctor, moderate exercise and activity can help combat fatigue, maintain muscle strength that can be diminished by surgery and other treatments, decrease anxiety, reduce feelings of depression, and help maintain a positive body image. Some hospitals are incorporating exercise classes, including yoga, chair aerobics, and personal training, all facilitated by specially trained experts. If you investigate local exercise programs, either through your hospital, a local gym, physical therapist, or community group, be sure someone who has experience with medical patients leads the programs. The cost of such services and programs varies. However, community groups such as senior centers, Gilda's Club, and the American Cancer Society sometimes sponsor exercise activities for free. It is crucial that you undergo any exercise routine safely so that you avoid injury and benefit from the exercise. You can also increase activity in your everyday life, such as walking more or taking the stairs at the hospital instead of the elevator, even if you have the energy for just one flight. One patient who was having a hard time with fatigue due to his chemotherapy and radiation felt that walking his hallway several times a day kept his body working and helped keep his mental strength as well. Being active includes fun things too, like going shopping, walking the dog, or playing with the kids. Keep it fun!

Pati's Comment:

Try to live as normal a life as possible, eat as well as you can, exercise, and reach out to family and friends. Most importantly, find a hobby that you enjoy. I find when I garden or work on arts and crafts projects, it takes my mind off my troubles.

Denial works both ways. Many people use the word denial, and they typically refer to it as a negative way to cope. However, denial can, in fact, be a useful coping technique, serving as a defense mechanism to shield you temporarily from emotions. Denial can help you avoid thoughts or emotions that would be too much for you to handle at one time. For example, Jack (mentioned in Question 76) used denial; it protected him from overwhelming emotions at the time of his initial diagnosis when he was making important treatment decisions when the reality of his colorectal cancer diagnosis did not yet seem real to him. However, his use of denial did not work well for him over the long haul when the reality sank in and he experienced his hidden emotions. Jack's situation illustrates a good point: Denial can be useful, but when it compromises your ability to cope, contradicts medical advice, or is extreme (to the point where you deny you even have cancer, for instance), it can lead to higher stress—particularly since people who deny the problem are less likely to solve it or ask for help when needed.

Prepare yourself. Patients often describe the time before surgery or chemotherapy and radiation therapy as a particularly stressful time. They may fear that the cancer is still growing in their bodies. Some people may demand radical treatment prematurely as a result of this stress. Furthermore, patients often misunderstand chemotherapy and radiation therapy, and this misunderstanding can cause extreme fear and dread in some patients. For example, some people assume that they will be very sick (including nausea, diarrhea, and so on), be in pain, and/or lose their hair. True, you may experience one or more of these symptoms, but new cancer treatments and medications that control side effects enable patients to better tolerate radiation therapy and chemotherapy. Many people experience few or no side effects, and others have more, but they continue to maintain an active lifestyle with minor changes to their daily activities. Talk to a former patient whose treatment was similar to yours; he/she may give you some useful tips on how to manage treatments. If you plan to have chemotherapy or radiation therapy, you may consider going to the treatment area(s) before starting treatment in order to familiarize yourself with the environment. Sometimes, it helps to actually see the treatment areas, making them seem less mysterious and making it easier for you to visualize the future—making it less "unknown." Most importantly, speak with your doctor or nurse to get correct information on what to expect from your type of treatment, including possible side effects and how you can prevent or treat them.

Pati's Comment:

Learn what the possible side effects of your treatment are so you will be prepared to act quickly. It took a while to find the right nausea prevention regime for me, but there are several to try. It was finally decided that I had anticipatory chemo anxiety, so Ativan™ [a medication to help reduce symptoms of anxiety] was added and helped both with anxiety and nausea. The most important tip is to chill your mouth about 15 minutes prior to, during, and after 5-FU; this prevents the chemo from surging to the delicate mouth membranes and causing mouth ulcers.

Relax. Relaxation techniques can reduce distress during certain treatments (such as chemo or radiation). Relaxation has also helped people reduce pain. Start simply by using self-taught relaxation techniques, such as simple deep breathing techniques, which can be very effective. Bring calm music CDs or tapes with you to your treatments or hospital stay (which also may be used to drown out the snoring patient next to you!). If you would like further guidance in using more advanced relaxation techniques, such as **hypnosis** or **progressive relaxation**, you can ask your physician, nurse, or social worker for a referral to licensed practitioners of yoga, massage, relaxation training, hypnosis, reflexology, and other methods of complementary therapies. Some hospitals and private centers provide comprehensive services that can work in conjunction with your medical treatment. No matter what you choose to do, discuss it first with your medical team to prevent complications. For example, some types of touch therapy, such as massage, may not be recommended by doctors if a person has metastases in his or her bones or certain other conditions.

Hypnosis

A type of therapy, led by a trained professional, that helps people focus on a specific issue or sensation with the intention of treating a certain problem, such as pain or stress.

Progressive relaxation

A method of stress reduction in which a person can focus on breathing and on relaxing body parts individually to gradually become more relaxed and less stressed.

Be in the moment and problem solve. Focus on one day at a time, one moment at a time, and solving one problem at a time. Try to move beyond thinking about the past, "what-ifs," and "whys." Instead, focus on the present and about how you are going to cope with the current problems, here and now. In other words, be in the moment. If you are feeling happy and calm, allow yourself to sit and enjoy this feeling. Whenever you are feeling distressed, identify what you are experiencing physically and emotionally. This will help you begin to focus on identifying the problem and to help solve it. If you are already on "overload," step back a moment and identify what you were thinking about before you felt overwhelmed. Second, identify your feelings. For example, do you feel regret or frustration at not being able to do what you want or believe you need? Next, problem solve by prioritizing your commitments according to their importance and according to other factors, such as your energy levels and other limits. By breaking down surmounting obligations, you will take control, be less overwhelmed, and reduce negative feelings.

Maintain hope. No matter what comes your way, try to maintain hope. Hope for what you feel is vital in your life. Many people hope for doing something special they have planned with family and friends. Others find hope in spiritual and religious realms. Identify what you hope for, even though this may change over time. Keep this thing in mind because it will help you to remember what you are living for.

Laugh. Despite the seriousness of their cancer diagnosis, many patients and their family members find that humor is crucial to their coping. Do not forget to laugh. More importantly, do not forget how to laugh. Humor and laughter can defuse tense situations and can be good stress relievers. Find humor and laughter in different places: identify a particularly funny person in your life and spend time with him or her, go to a comedic movie, or even go to a live comedy show. If you find it hard to do such things, do still try them, and remember to focus on the moment as much as you can. It will help you enjoy the jokes and laugh, lighten your mood, and take your mind off the more serious things for a while.

82. I have been using the suggested coping techniques, but I still feel down most of the time, and I constantly worry about my cancer despite the fact that I was diagnosed almost 2 months ago. What should I do? Can counseling help?

Despite using adaptive coping skills, many people still find that further guidance is helpful. A good place to start finding help is your medical team (your doctor, nurse, social worker, or chaplain). Sometimes people feel much better after a single conversation about their feelings, particularly because feeling depressed and anxious is common among people with cancer. You may feel relieved to know that others have experienced similar feelings. However, if you still feel that you need help after an initial discussion or you think you may be suffering from depression or anxiety (see Question 80), you may want to explore additional methods for getting support. Many places provide support and counseling. You may want to meet with your hospital social worker or contact your local chapter of the American Cancer Society to point you in the right direction.

Counseling. Many people find that individual or family counseling (or -therapy) helps them cope with the emotional aspects of having cancer. Professionals are trained to help people feel their best, both psychologically and emotionally. Below is a brief list of the most common mental health professionals:

Licensed Clinical Social Workers: Commonly have a LSW, LCSW or LMSW. Trained clinicians, usually with at least a master's degree (MSW, MSSW) and additional training or expertise in their specialty. Clinical social workers practice in a variety of settings, including hospitals, counseling or mental health centers, and private practice. Depending on their expertise, they are able to diagnose and treat psychological problems using counseling. They are also trained in more general counseling to help you through difficult time periods in your life, with or without an exact psychological diagnosis.

Psychologists: Have a PhD or a PsyD. Psychologists can also diagnose and treat psychological issues and are usually trained in specific theories of therapy, such as psychodynamic, interpersonal or cognitive/behavioral therapies. Neither psychologists nor social workers can prescribe medications, but they can refer you to a medical doctor (your primary physician, your oncologist, or a psychiatrist), who can evaluate your need for medications to treat depression, anxiety, or other mental health problems.

Psychiatrists: Medical doctors (MDs) who specialize in diagnosing and treating psychiatric disorders by prescribing medications and/or providing therapy. They are experts on the physiological aspects of psychological problems, such as depression and anxiety.

Other mental health professionals: Psychiatric nurses, master's-level counselors, pastoral counselors, alternative/complementary medicine practitioners, and other mental health professionals can also provide certain types of counseling and anxiety-reduction techniques. As with any other professionals, be sure to investigate their qualifications and experience.

Questions to ask a mental health professional:

1. What is your training and are you licensed in this state?
2. Do you have experience helping people with cancer (or family members of people with cancer)?
3. What do you charge? Do you accept my insurance policy?
4. How often and where can I see you (in a private office, in the hospital)?
5. What do I do about an after-hours emergency? Whom should I call?

Groups. People with cancer and their family members often find that talking to other people who are also affected by cancer helps them understand that they are not alone. They often learn new ways of coping and are relieved to be able to discuss their concerns openly with others who have had the same experiences and who understand. There are different types of support groups. Some agencies, such as Cancer Care, Inc., offer traditional groups as well as innovative groups that are conducted on the Internet and on the telephone. These groups are particularly helpful to people who are not comfortable meeting many new people, simply do not feel well enough to travel from their homes, and/or live too far away from group meetings.

Professionals facilitate some groups, while cancer survivors or family members of patients (for groups intended for family) lead other groups. *Therapy groups* are intended to treat a specific psychological problem, such as clinical depression, and are usually led by a mental health professional. *Support groups* focus on sharing experiences, providing emotional support to people as well as helping to reduce distress and relieve isolation. *Educational groups*, on the other hand, are used to provide information to a large group of people, such as different coping tools, relaxation training, ostomy care, and management of medical issues. This kind of group focuses less on people sharing their feelings and may be good for those who do not want to attend a traditional support group but would still benefit from interaction with others. Support and education-focused groups can be led by a variety of professionals and volunteers. For help locating support groups, speak with your medical team or social worker or consult our resource list at the back of this book. The American Cancer Society can be particularly helpful in directing you to local groups.

Questions to ask when investigating a group:

1. Does a professional lead this group? Or does a volunteer facilitate it?
2. Do I have to commit to a certain number of sessions?
3. What date does the group start? How long is each session?
4. Where does the group meet, and may I have directions to the meeting?
5. Is there a cost to attend this group? If so, do you accept my insurance?
6. What topics are covered? Is this a group for people with specific problems (depression, anxiety)?
7. Does this group focus on a specific cancer diagnosis?

Patient volunteers. Patient-to-patient programs (or "buddy" programs) also exist to help you cope with your cancer. Most commonly these programs organize patient volunteers (often those who completed treatment several years before) who interact with people who are currently diagnosed with cancer. Volunteers can provide a variety of support services, ranging from basic advice to more complex problems, such as coping with a new diagnosis. The volunteers can suggest strategies for getting through surgery, chemotherapy and/or radiation treatments, for dealing with common frustrations of being part of the medical system, and so on. Most importantly, former colorectal patients provide hope to people who are currently battling cancer. Particularly if you are not interested in a support group, you may find talking with an individual volunteer helpful.

1. Hospital-based volunteers: Many hospitals and many doctors have formal and informal ways of connecting you with former patients for support. Ask your doctor, nurse, or social worker for information.
2. National organizations: If you do not find a patient volunteer program at your hospital, contact Cancer Care, Inc., the Colon Cancer Alliance, or the Cancer Hope Network.

83. Should I consider using medications to help my depression and anxiety?

Medications are helpful to some patients suffering from depression, anxiety, and other high levels of distress. Depression and anxiety result from physiological changes in the brain and can be helped with medications such as antidepressants and anti-anxiety prescriptions. Sometimes people are reluctant to take such medication because they are afraid that it means that they are unbalanced, the pills will change their personality, they will become addicted, or their doctor will treat them differently (or think that they are weak). Some people also believe, erroneously, that such medications will make their tumors grow faster. Keep in mind that medications merely alleviate the problem for which they were prescribed, with the intention of making the patient more comfortable and in control. Taking a prescription to reduce your distress does not mean that you are "going crazy." Some people are hesitant to try these medications because of the stigma they believe is attached to them; many of these folks who later take the medications wonder why they waited so long. They feel so much better and are better able to cope and enjoy life. Often these medications are most effective when combined with counseling and/or group support.

Although drug therapy can be helpful, these medications are not for everyone. They are not magic pills that will take away all your problems; the issues -troubling you will still exist, but the medications just may make them easier for you to manage. You need to make the right decision for you. In addition, these medications sometimes take several weeks to start working and sometimes produce side effects. You should discuss the pros and cons of each medicine you take with your doctor. Sometimes people have to try different brands or types of medication to find the one that works the best. Any physician, such as your primary doctor or oncologist, can prescribe such medicines; however, you may consider an initial evaluation and/or regular follow-up with a psychiatrist.

84. Ever since I first suspected I had cancer, I have had recurring thoughts and dreams about death, including how my own death will be. Sometimes, I think of frightening things, while other times it is peaceful. Is this normal? Is thinking about death bad luck? Does it mean that I am going to die of this cancer?

When someone is faced with the news that he or she has cancer, frequent thoughts of death are common. Death is something that, at least in the United States and many other cultures, people often try to forget about; they simply deny that it exists. A cancer diagnosis cuts right through this denial and fears of mortality flood through. Some people are prepared for this realization; others are not. For those who are not prepared, this may be the first time in their lives that they have truly realized they are mortal. Thoughts of death may include the following:

- Thinking about your own impending death and what it will be like
- Remembering past experiences with death and losses
- Paying more attention to death in the news or books
- Talking more about it to family, friends, or religious leaders
- Worrying about pain and other medical aspects about the dying process

Ironically, understanding your beliefs about death can be helpful to your coping. In order to understand yourself better, pay attention to when you think about death, what you specifically think about, and how you feel about these thoughts. If you want to discuss these issues, find someone with whom you can talk openly about death and dying. If people close to you (family, friends) misinterpret discussions of death as you are "giving up" or find them too much to handle, find someone more objective to speak to, such as a religious leader, your doctor or nurse, or a counselor. Additionally, becoming more aware of your fears and intentions can be helpful when you are speaking to your loved ones about your wishes regarding end-of-life care (see Questions 98 and 99). Thinking about death does not make it come faster, nor is it bad luck.

If you find yourself thinking about death and dying for long periods of time (for most of the day, many days in a row), or if you think about taking steps to end your life, contact your doctor, mental health professional, or 911 immediately. Depression and other psychological issues can make thoughts of death overwhelming. Additionally, people who are experiencing various physical symptoms or side effects may misinterpret these experiences, believing that they are actually dying (when, in fact, they are not). Pain and other factors altering quality of life are common predecessors to thoughts of wanting to die. However, when these medical problems are solved, thoughts or wishes of death usually subside as well. Therefore, if you are comfortable, talk about your thoughts and feelings about dying with your family and with the medical team. Sharing your feelings can be helpful to you and will also help your family and team to understand you better and to help you in your time of distress.

FAMILY AND FRIENDS

85. Whom do I tell about my cancer diagnosis, what do I tell them, and how will they react?

Some people do not tell anyone anything (sometimes not even their spouses) about the cancer diagnosis, whereas others tell the world everything (literally, by writing books about their experiences). Disclosure is a highly personal decision. Telling no one can lead to lack of support and isolation. If you are having concerns about disclosure, perhaps the best way to determine what is right for you is to start talking to people selectively, including your very close family and friends who can be helpful to you during the initial diagnosis, information gathering, and discussions with the medical team. These people can be the biggest help to you in this phase. As you learn more about your cancer, prognosis, and treatment plan, you may be prepared to tell more people and to know what to tell them.

What you tell others will depend on how comfortable you feel discussing your medical issues. Some people feel stigmatized about having cancer. Discussions about colorectal cancer, the rectum, the anus, and bowel movements are not typical dinner conversation. The first step to moving beyond the stigma is for you to accept the diagnosis yourself. After you feel more comfortable talking about your diagnosis with others, they will usually feel more comfortable discussing it as well.

You can become more comfortable in many ways. First, learn about your cancer, such as where in the body it is located and about the functions of that body part. Second, practice talking about your diagnosis with close, trusted friends and family. See how they react and what questions they have. Often, knowing what other people think or might ask helps you prepare yourself for what to tell other people. Third, if you feel comfortable and choose to tell other people, start talking about your diagnosis more openly. If it fits with your personality, humor is often a good icebreaker and can make you and others feel more at ease.

Remember, people have their own conceptions about cancer, including colorectal cancer. People's reactions may surprise you. For some, talking about cancer elicits fear and misunderstanding, and they may want to avoid the topic. Some people erroneously believe that cancer is contagious or that cancer is always terminal. Some people with cancer feel rejected by others' unintentional reactions, sometimes from close friends who do not call anymore or do not want to socialize. On the other hand, other friends, or even distant acquaintances, may offer their support; old friendships can grow and new friendships can bloom.

Some people may be very interested in your diagnosis, treatment, and even prognosis. For these reactions, provide only as much information as you feel comfortable providing—don't feel pressured to divulge too much. They may also want to share their own experiences with cancer or information that they think will be helpful to you. You may find advice and sharing helpful, particularly in the beginning. Sometimes this information can be confusing, particularly when the information is irrelevant to your situation or when it is upsetting. If you start to feel overwhelmed, simply tell people that you appreciate their concern, but you feel better discussing your medical concerns solely with your doctor. You may hear of, or know of, other people diagnosed with cancer, maybe even colorectal cancer, who are not faring well medically. Remember, however, that every person is different, every cancer is different, and every person's response to treatment is unique.

Most people will be supportive and sensitive to your needs and offer support. Be prepared to accept such offers, and do not be afraid to ask for specific help, such as driving your children to their activities, preparing food, helping with laundry and cleaning, or just doing something fun together. People with whom you share your diagnosis are often relieved when you ask for specific help as it takes pressure off of them to try to figure out how to help. They want to feel useful and be involved. Furthermore, by accepting help you may feel less stressed by having fewer drains on your energy.

Your cancer will affect your entire family and those around you. These people closest to you may express a mixture of negative and positive reactions, some of which may be similar to your own thoughts and feelings. For example, it is normal for your loved ones to sometimes feel angry that you have cancer, think that it is unfair, or feel helpless because they cannot protect you from this cancer or its effects. However, just as you find support from them, they may find more open communication helpful, too.

86. My spouse/partner was recently diagnosed with colorectal cancer, and I am feeling overwhelmed. How can I "be strong" and supportive for my loved one while continuing to cope with my own reactions to this diagnosis?

After his wife was diagnosed with cancer, one husband said, "I feel like I am a passenger in a car on a dangerous, icy road. My wife is driving and she is in ultimately in control of crucial decisions that will affect both of us, and I am fearful of what will happen." Just as patients feel a loss of control when they are diagnosed with a medical illness, caregivers also often feel a loss of control. As a spouse, you are an observer of what is happening, but you are also profoundly affected by your partner's reactions and decisions.

Caregivers also often feel a loss of control.

As you are coping with your own reactions to the diagnosis of your loved one, you are also being expected to perform new functions that may be new to you. Your role as caregiver can jump between being a partner and acting like a nurse, a housekeeper, a cook, a psychologist, a chauffeur, a secretary, or others. Sometimes you may not know which role to play at any given time. As a partner, you will probably share a large burden of caregiving responsibilities. Emotionally, spouses report sometimes feeling helpless and feel that they cannot do enough. You may experience feelings similar to that of the patient, such as depression, sadness, anxiety, and fear. Your life will be disrupted, so understand that these adjustments represent significant changes, and allow yourself time to come to grips with them.

These changes can cause conflicts between you and your spouse, particularly if you are not prepared to talk about these issues as they arise, or if you have had relationship problems before the diagnosis of cancer. For many couples, communication can use fine-tuning, even before a diagnosis of cancer. If you need some direction on how to begin more open communication about your spouse's diagnosis, start by asking your partner questions about how he/she is feeling (both physically and emotionally), and how you can help. For example, you may ask:

- How are you holding up?
- Tell me—what is this really like for you?
- I notice that you have been quiet lately; do you mind telling me what you are thinking about?
- I will try to be here for you in any way I can. Would you give me some pointers on ways I can help?

You may also want to express your thoughts and feelings to your spouse. Couples often want to protect each other from their feelings, and in essence, put up an emotional wall. If you take the lead, your spouse may feel that it is OK to share as well. However, remember that you do not need to share everything, all the time, particularly if you are not comfortable talking about your feelings. Find what works for you—do not force yourself, or your spouse, to talk.

In addition to communicating feelings and needs, you may also consider doing the following to help your partner, depending on how he or she is feeling:

- Try not to let the topic of cancer dominate all conversation—talk about other things.
- Live life with your spouse. Do enjoyable activities together.
- Buy a thoughtful gift as a token of your feelings.
- Take on the "Public Relations" role by communicating to other people how your spouse is doing.
- Touch your spouse. Touch is an important part of intimacy and reassurance, particularly when words are not enough. Touch is also calming.
- Allow your spouse to feel what he or she is feeling; if your spouse is feeling down, ask why he or she is feeling that way, instead of instantly trying to "fix" the problem or pressuring your spouse to be more positive.
- Do gently remind your spouse about positive aspects of life, such as people who love him or her or upcoming enjoyable events, like a wedding or party.
- Help your spouse feel less dependent and more in control. Reassure your spouse that you are fulfilling your role as caregiver out of love, and try to help your spouse maintain as much control as possible by continuing to participate in household decisions, making social plans, or doing other activities independently according to how he/she is feeling.

Tip: If you are interested in improving communication, keep in mind that "forcing" your spouse to talk, or suddenly changing your methods of communication, may not bring about your intended result of better communication. Instead, try asking open-ended questions and listen to what your spouse says. Listening is as important as talking (sometimes even more so!).

Listening is as important as talking.

In addition to focusing on your spouse's needs, make your needs a priority as well. You may choose to talk to your spouse or someone else, such as a good friend, family member, or maybe a spouse of another patient who is going through similar experiences. You may meet other spouses at various medical appointment waiting rooms or other places, such as support groups. If you are having problems coping, find a professional to talk to or find a family/caregiver support group in your area. And, of primary importance, take time out for yourself, away from the cancer and the hospital. Take a respite; ask another family member/caregiver or friend to step in to help if needed. If you do not take care of yourself, you will not be at your best for your partner.

87. I have two young children. I don't want to tell them about my diagnosis and surgery because I don't want to upset them. I can barely handle this myself, so how can they cope with it? Should I tell them about my cancer, and if so, how much? What if they ask if I am going to die?

Telling your children about your cancer diagnosis is one of the most difficult issues you may have to face as a parent. Some people are reluctant to tell their children, whereas others want to be as open as possible. Research and the professional experience of oncology counselors indicate that telling children the truth from the beginning generally leads to better adjustment. However, as their parent, you are the expert on

Telling children the truth from the beginning generally leads to better adjustment.

your children, and you should keep them involved as much as you and they feel comfortable. If you are a grandparent, or other family member, you may also find the following information helpful.

Obviously, the ages of children affect what type and how much information they can comprehend. For example, a 4-year-old will not understand as much detail as a 10-year-old, nor will a 10-year-old understand as much as a teenager. However, the following guidelines may be helpful and, unless otherwise stated, are good things to keep in mind for all age groups of children.

- Children have a good sense for what is going on with you and your family; they often sense subtle changes as well as obvious ones (including concerns about hospital bills, overhearing you or a family member on the phone). Therefore, they may know about your diagnosis anyway, and maybe they should hear it from you—the earlier, the better. This is a time to develop trust with your child regarding your diagnosis and treatment.
- Because every type of cancer is different, and each person's treatment is individually tailored, you need to give your children the opportunity to ask about your cancer and treatments so that they do not get misinformation (from the Internet, friends, or other children).
- If they have known someone else who died from cancer, you need to reassure them that this is not necessarily going to happen to you. Give them age-appropriate specifics about your cancer and treatment, including how your cancer is different.
- Children, too, often blame themselves for things, including a parent's cancer diagnosis. Many children create fantasies to explain things. They might think that you got cancer because they were not doing well in school or because they shouted something at you or secretly wished that something bad would happen to you

the last time they were punished. You may be surprised at what they may be thinking. Ask them. They need reassurance that they are not the cause of the cancer.

- Conversely, because children often think that they did something to cause the cancer, they sometimes think that they have the power to make it go away. A youngster sometimes becomes the "model child" and tries to do everything right. A teenager may suddenly become overly helpful around the house or become a "substitute parent." Sometimes parents mistake this exemplary behavior to mean that their child is coping well. Being the perfect child can be a tremendous burden for your child because of the feelings of responsibility that this method of coping entails; children may fear that they will "mess up" and make you worse, or if you experience a complication, they may feel guilty that they did not try hard enough to be perfect.
- Children often focus on how cancer will affect their lives, occasionally appearing selfish and expressing anger and frustration. Teenagers and children may resent being asked to help with household duties to help a sick parent. Try to be patient with a child who expresses these feelings and to understand without judgment (which can be difficult). Attempt to find solutions, such as temporarily hiring a housekeeper or asking family or neighbors to help with household functions so that household routines are less disrupted.
- Children of all ages often ask the "hard" questions that adults have learned not to blurt out. For example, sometimes, the first question out of a younger child's mouth after talking with his/her parent who has cancer is "Are you doing to die?" This is the hard one; not only can it bring up tremendous feelings of fear and anxiety in you, but it is also the time when most parents want to reassure their child (and themselves) that everything is going to be OK and that, of course, Mommy or Daddy will not die, will never die. However, this is simply not

true. Just as flowers and pets will die, everyone dies at some point. It is important that you reassure your child, but do not misrepresent the truth. You can say something like, "Yes, I do have cancer in my colon. However, I am getting the best treatment and seeing the best doctors who are going to try everything to fight this cancer. Everyone dies someday, but I am going to battle this cancer with all my might."

- Your children may react differently after they discuss your cancer with you and your family. Some children, especially very young children, can digest only bits of information at a time. They may not ask questions initially, so make sure that the "big talk" is not just a one-time thing. Continue to check in with your children to see how they are doing and to tell them how you are doing, too. However, if they do not want to talk, do not push them. Instead, tell them that they can ask you any question they like, which gives them control. Remember that if you have more than one child, each one may react differently.
- The word "cancer" is an abstract term that is often hard for children to understand, which can lead to increased fear and misunderstanding. Showing children age-appropriate pictures and diagrams of the body, including where the cancer is located—or especially for younger children, allowing them to draw pictures of it themselves—will help them conceptualize the cancer. One 6-year-old girl drew a picture of her father with a big black dot on his "tummy," representing the cancer. This picture made it much easier for her to visualize and talk about the cancer with her parents.
- Some children become very involved and interested in cancer and treatment. They may even want to attend appointments or visit you at the hospital. Allowing them to attend an appointment (after first discussing this with your physician and establishing guidelines) may be a good way for them to be reassured

and have the opportunity to ask questions. However, it is important not to overwhelm them with information; otherwise, this meeting may make them more anxious, having an effect that is the opposite of what you intended. Children who want to come with you to chemotherapy or visit the hospital should be prepared beforehand. Tell them about the treatments and about what they might see (including tubes, other sick patients, and so on). Taking a picture of yourself in treatment can also help them visualize what they might see before they arrive. Some children want to learn about all the tubes, stitches, and other accessories of treatment. Feel free to give them as much information as you, and they, feel comfortable with. Remember, you are the expert on your child, so pay attention to your instincts and stop when you feel they have experienced enough.

- Take steps to ensure that significant adults (such as caregivers, close family, teachers, and school counselors) around your child are providing consistent messages. You may want to tell these adults generally what you are going through medically and what your child already knows. These people will be able to provide support to your child and also notify you if they have concerns about how your child is coping.
- Providing physical reassurance, such as hugs and touch, is important to you and your child, especially infants or toddlers, for whom modes of communication are limited. You may not be able to play "rough" with your children immediately after surgery or because of fatigue, so explain this to your children and substitute other activities and forms of physical connection (such as sitting close together watching a video or reading together). You do not want them to mistake a lack of physical attention as rejection.
- Continue (as much as possible) with precancer routines and disciplinary actions. This may be difficult because

you have demands on your time, but try to allow your child to remain in his or her activities, see friends, and get up in the morning and go to bed at the same times. Some parents want to be more indulgent and some more strict, however, this is not going to make your child cope any better. Consistency communicates security to children.

- If you are unsure about how to talk to your child or have concerns about how he or she is coping with the diagnosis, speak to a social worker or counselor who specializes in helping children of a parent with cancer. If your children are in school, talking with their teachers and/or school counselor can be helpful too. There are also many resources that may help, including "How to Help Children Through a Parent's Serious Illness" by Kathleen McCue, and other resources in the back of this book (see the Appendix on page 215). If you have concerns about how your children are coping with your diagnosis, you can investigate counseling for your children or groups intended specially for children coping with a parent diagnosed with cancer.

Tip: Be honest and consistent, and reassure your child that your cancer is no one's fault.

88. Now that I have completed cancer treatment, how do I get on with my life?

Advances in the early diagnosis and treatment of colorectal cancer are increasing the number of people who survive the disease. However, this also means that more people with a personal history of cancer may need input about putting their cancer behind them and moving on to live life fully again. This may seem easy, but for some people, it is not. They may ask themselves, "Isn't this what I have dreamt about since my diagnosis? Shouldn't I be grateful for surviving cancer?" Additionally, the following issues may arise in the post-treatment phase of your cancer recovery:

- Management of follow-up medical appointments
- Fear of cancer recurrence
- Changed self-esteem and self-image
- Legal and financial issues after diagnosis (initiating a new job search or writing the right résumé)
- Concern about possible genetic predisposition of cancer in family members
- Concern about future medical issues, follow-ups, and screening
- Leading a healthy lifestyle, including exercising, stopping smoking, and changing dietary habits
- Unresolved life issues that were postponed because of diagnosis and treatment (such as marriage or separation, having children, or changing careers)
- Long-term treatment side effects, such as scars, ostomy, infertility, and sexual issues

Often, techniques used for coping with your cancer will help you develop a broader understanding of your life that includes all of your experiences, including surviving cancer. However, sometimes after treatment, survivors experience new problems coping and investigate new avenues to help themselves. For some who coped well during the whole diagnosis and treatment phase, the realization of the cancer experience hits them long after the ordeal is over. If you experience some problems moving forward, you may want to find a support group, another survivor, or a mental health professional to help you understand and manage these issues as you work toward restoring your quality of life.

Techniques used for coping with your cancer will help you develop a broader understanding of your life.

MANAGING POSSIBLE PHYSICAL CHANGES

89. I have heard that I may experience physical changes after surgery. Will any of these affect my sexuality or fertility? Will I become impotent? Why is this risk higher after surgery for rectal cancer than after colon cancer?

The nerves that control the sexual organs lie next to the rectum. During surgery for rectal cancer, these nerves can be damaged, resulting in physical sexual changes. These complications are extremely rare with regular colon surgery because these nerves are outside of the normal operating area for colon surgery.

Men who have undergone rectal cancer surgery and have suffered nerve injury may experience two different types of sexual dysfunction: (1) they may lose the ability to maintain an erection (**impotence**), or (2) they may become infertile but still remain able to perform sexual intercourse. In the second case, the ability to perform sexual intercourse remains intact, however, infertility (the inability to conceive) can occur.

Impotence

Inability to maintain an erection that is sufficient to engage in sexual activity.

The radical surgery performed for lower rectal cancers has improved recently so that such complications are uncommon during routine surgery. The incidence of impotence for all male patients ranges from 10% to 30%. This statistic includes individuals with large, advanced tumors; older patients, who may already suffer from impotence; and those undergoing APR (complete removal of the anus, the rectum, and the surrounding muscles of the anal canal) rather than low anterior resection (removal of the lower portion of the rectum). If these groups were not included in the tallying of impotence after surgery, the incidence of impotence would likely be even less. Fortunately, there are many treatments for these postoperative complications, and you can be referred by your physician to a specialist if this rare situation occurs.

Sexual changes in women after rectal surgery are less clearly defined. Some women may experience vaginal dryness and pain during intercourse. These problems seem to occur less frequently than those faced by men, and they can often be treated easily with topical creams and lubricants.

Sometimes radiation therapy, chemotherapy and certain surgeries can cause infertility for both men and women. To be successful, it is often important that steps are taken before treatment begins for most kinds of fertility options, such as sperm-banking or harvesting eggs. New fertility improvement options are also available, particularly for women, such as preservation of ovarian tissue removed before treatment which can later be implanted back into the body after cancer therapy is finished. Eggs are then harvested and fertilized, with the hope of creating embryos. Other types of state-of-the-art research is being conducted assessing methods of preserving fertility among cancer survivors at the Center for Reproductive Medicine and Infertility in New York City, and many other clinical/research centers (see Question 100 for contact information).

In addition to exploring the medical and technology options, also be sure to investigate insurance coverage and the costs associated with such fertility treatments. There are now organizations advocating for better insurance coverage and possible financial assistance to young adult cancer patients for fertility treatments, such as Fertilehope (see Question 100 for contact information).

90. What techniques can I use to deal with sexual changes associated with colorectal cancer?

As a person moves beyond the initial phase of diagnosis and making treatment decisions, questions regarding other important aspects of a person's life become increasingly important. Often, such concerns focus on intimacy, sexuality, and sexual side effects during and after diagnosis and treatment. For some people, however, sex is a difficult topic to talk about, both with your partner and with the medical team. However, open communication can be an important factor in maintaining or regaining your sexuality. If you are having surgery, you may experience a decrease in your sex drive before surgery because you may be preoccupied with your upcoming treatment and, similarly, during your recuperation. Afterward, you may experience body changes, including scars and/or an ostomy. Also, depending on the type of treatment you undergo, different types of sexual problems can result (see Question 89). Some people feel embarrassed about these alterations to their body, particularly when they first get out of surgery. With time, you can become accustomed to possible body changes, particularly with assistance from medical professionals (including your **enterostomal specialist** if you have an ostomy) and by discussing your concerns with the team and your partner. Intimacy will not hurt your incision (once it has healed) or your ostomy.

Enterostomal specialist

Usually a nurse with special training in ostomy care, including coping with body changes after surgery.

If you are experiencing sexual changes, and these changes are important to you, this may be a good time to think creatively about sex and intimacy. Touching, caressing, oral and finger stimulation, and use of sexual paraphernalia are sometimes as arousing and stimulating as traditional sexual intercourse (or more so for some people). If you are concerned about your partner seeing your ostomy pouch or scars, wear lingerie or a T-shirt. As you start to experiment, you may find new ways of pleasing your partner and new activities that you enjoy, too. Often, couples experience a resurgence in loving feelings toward one another when they are faced with cancer; focus on these feelings during lovemaking and sexual practice.

If you are single, you may be particularly sensitive to initiating intimate relationships with new partners. Beginning sexual practice will take time and each situation is different so listen to yourself and follow your instincts. Also, keep in mind that sexual adjustment for all colorectal patients starts with being informed and with learning good communication. If you continue to have questions or experience problems, you may want to contact a physician or a therapist who specializes in treating sexual issues.

91. I recently had surgery, and I have an ostomy. Before surgery, I didn't realize how hard this was going to be. Now, the medical team expects me to learn to care for this "thing"... and I don't even want to look at it, let alone do all the rest. How do I get beyond this dread and fear?

Cancer, surgery, and treatment are hard enough to deal with; an ostomy brings unique concerns, and you will need assistance coping with body changes and ostomy care. Having an ostomy sometimes increases the anxiety, fear, and shame that some people with colorectal cancer feel. People do not think much about "natural" body functions, including bowel movements—that is, until these functions are about to be changed or disrupted. Some people are hesitant about the possibility of an ostomy, and they need extra time to decide to undergo surgery and seek reassurance (see Question 93). However, people generally adjust well after surgery. Other people may underestimate the challenges they face when adjusting to a colostomy or ileostomy until after the surgery. Complicating matters, just when the reality of the surgery, the ostomy, and its implications are sinking in, patients may feel pressure from doctors, nurses, and family to accept and care for the ostomy.

Take steps to prevent yourself from becoming overwhelmed right from the beginning. Meet with the ostomy nurse specialist as soon as possible, and establish realistic goals for yourself. If you are having problems adjusting, ask yourself why and discuss these issues with the ostomy specialist and/or surgeon. These meetings will bring you closer to independently caring for your ostomy.

Pace yourself.

Keep in mind that your psychological and physical adjustment to your new ostomy is not going to occur overnight. Pace yourself. You will most likely have a home care ostomy specialist or other nurse professional visit you after you are discharged from the hospital to provide additional instruction and support. You may find that attending at least one ostomy education or support group is helpful (contact the United Ostomy Association of America or your doctor, nurse, or social worker for referrals). Gather written materials from your medical team and other reputable organizations to reinforce the training. And, at follow-up appointments, discuss how you are doing with the ostomy, including any questions you may have about its care and your adjustment. If you find it helpful, make arrangements to see the enterostomal therapist to provide more intensive ongoing advice and support.

Discuss any initial restrictions after surgery with your doctor (such as heavy lifting or impact sports). Other than these restrictions, you should be able to resume familiar activities as you recuperate with few, if any, physical consequences. You can still perform all your daily activities and participate in physical sports with an ostomy—you can play golf, tennis, ski, and even swim. In fact, limitations to your activities will most likely come from your self-imposed restrictions that result from your emotional adjustment to the colostomy. Some people avoid social activities, sports such as swimming, or sexual experiences because they are afraid that people will see, smell, or somehow know that they have an ostomy. As you become more familiar with the ostomy and its care, you will realize that people are unlikely to know about your ostomy unless you show or tell them. The ostomy bag is made of materials that adhere closely to your body, making it invisible under almost all types of clothing (see Question 92). Furthermore, taking simple steps can prevent smell and gas. Become active in your ostomy care, and with a little patience, you will soon find that you can live much like you did before your surgery.

92. Now that I am moving beyond the initial shock of having an ostomy, what are the basic things I need to know?

A stoma appliance (or ostomy appliance) is a device that collects the waste from an ostomy. It usually consists of two pieces: a faceplate (or "wafer") that is taped to the skin of a person's abdomen around the ostomy opening, and a separate plastic bag, or pouch, that collects the waste, although one-piece appliances do exist. During the course of the day, as the bag fills, it needs to be emptied. People who have colostomies usually need to empty the bag 2 to 3 times a day while people with ileostomies usually empty it more frequently because more waste tends to collect. A person can simply go to a restroom and empty the bag contents into the toilet.

Ostomy appliances come in all different shapes and sizes for a personalized fit. The opening on the adhesive faceplate is cut carefully to fit exactly around the stoma and reduce the risk of leakage and skin irritation. Some faceplates are a level circle, and others are curved, producing a better seal on flat stomas. Various skin protectants and cleaning materials are used to prepare the skin for the appliance. Bags also come in a variety of sizes. Some are clear plastic whereas others are colored and opaque (difficult to see through) and hide their contents. Special charcoal filters can be used to minimize the odor associated with stomal output. Although the plastic bag is emptied frequently during the day, the faceplate needs to be replaced only once approximately every 4 days. The appliance can get wet and so is worn during showers or baths without a problem.

Colostomy waste is mostly solid and can be controlled with a combination of diet and stoma techniques. For example, many people with colostomies are able to control their waste output with routine colostomy irrigation (rinsing). Colostomy irrigation is performed with an enema that is administered into the stoma. This is done at the same time every day, often first thing in the morning. This empties the end of the colon of waste and often takes only 15 to 30 minutes to perform. With this part of the colon emptied of stool, waste output is minimized during the day. Therefore, a colostomy bag may not be necessary, and either a smaller attachment can be used, or even just a gauze pad.

Ostomies are situated below the belly button and slightly to one side. This allows a small part of the intestine (a stoma) to be brought through the abdominal wall and limits hernia formation. The stoma is placed on top of the abdominal fat pad, making it easy to see and care for. Your surgeon will avoid locating it within the skin folds so that there can be maximum contact between the faceplate and the skin. Usually, the bag will fall below the pants line and can be easily hidden from view. Baggy clothes may be more convenient, as is the use of suspenders instead of a belt, for example.

If your surgeon has told you that you are likely to have an ostomy, you will likely be scheduled for a preoperative assessment by an enterostomal specialist (or ostomy nurse specialist). During evaluation, a site will be identified and marked on your abdomen so that the stoma will be placed in the best possible position on the body. After surgery, the enterostomal specialist will be a valuable resource for managing your stoma and helping you if you have any concerns. These specialists are also experts in selecting the correct appliances for you.

93. I think I would rather die than live with a permanent stoma. Can't I just let this disease take its natural course without subjecting myself to this treatment?

Kate's Comment:

I've met lots of ostomates, and they have helped me see that life with an ostomy can be very manageable. My mom's 1950-style colostomy, messy and difficult to manage, has been replaced with new surgical techniques, new and better ostomy appliances, and new ways of keeping the ostomy clean and emptied. My ostomate friends all urge getting good planning for placement of the stoma by having an experienced ostomy nurse measure you sitting and standing. They also tell me that support from others with ostomies and help from the ostomy nurses helps you learn to manage.

Being diagnosed with cancer is a tremendous burden on anyone, and your ability to cope with your feelings may be more difficult if you are told that a permanent or temporary stoma is necessary. Most people do not want to live with an ostomy, and some people may even consider not having the surgery or the stoma. If you are having this reaction, take a step back and review your decision-making process so that you can be sure that you are making the best decision for you. Weigh your values when making any treatment decision, including whether or not to have an ostomy. Some people who initially decline the ostomy procedure do later change their minds, after the initial shock and feelings subside. Sometimes taking the time to talk more to the surgeon or to other people who have been living with an ostomy can help ease this decision-making process.

When discussing the pros and cons with your surgeon, ask about the location and the stage of the tumor, and confirm the need for a colostomy. If an ostomy is indeed recommended, and you are still unsure of whether or not to proceed with surgery, make sure you are aware of the consequences. It is important that you understand that "letting nature take its course" does not necessarily mean you will slip gradually into a gentle death; not having the surgery can result in medical complications, including possible obstruction of the colon and tumor invasion of other organs, which can lower your quality of life. Refusing an ostomy may also hasten your death. Get a second opinion if you are still unsure. In fact, your insurance company may require a second opinion, so use this added information to help make the right medical decisions for you. Research your choice and take control over your decisions. Do keep in mind that over 60% of all patients with colorectal cancer survive. A stoma may represent a significant change in lifestyle, but it can be a means of survival. However, do not be pressured into having the surgery until you are comfortable with your decision. If you want more information on ostomies, support in adjusting to this type of surgery, or help making treatment decisions, refer to the Appendix on page 215.

WORK AND FINANCIAL ISSUES

94. Will I be able to continue working during radiation treatments and chemotherapy?

Kate's Comment:

I went back to work 3 weeks after my first surgery and about a month after the second one. I arranged weekly chemotherapy for the end of the week so I would have the weekend to recover. I arranged my office so I could have a nap in the afternoon. Other people in the office picked up pieces of work for me, and I tried to lighten my workload wherever I could. I scheduled my most difficult tasks for early morning when I felt rested and alert. While this was doable, I was exhausted most of the time. My weekends, when I could have spent time doing things I enjoyed, were spent in bed or on the sofa. Given another choice, if it were professionally and financially possible, I'd take the chemo treatment time for rest, recovery, and doing some of the things that make me the happiest.

The choice to continue working during treatments is a personal one. Radiation treatment sometimes requires being at the hospital or clinic up to an hour a day, and chemotherapy can also require regular visits to the hospital, posing a time constraint. Ideal times for treatment cannot always be coordinated with your work schedule. In addition, although the treatments themselves are usually painless, you may experience various side effects because of the toxic nature of the treatments. In other words, sometimes the substances or treatments that are given with the intent to kill your cancer can make you feel sick as well. For example, some patients experience diarrhea and fatigue. Although these symptoms can be minor, they can sometimes become more bothersome, particularly when radiation and chemotherapy are combined. Your choice of how much to work will need to be based on your type of work, the convenience of your hospital location to your daily activities, your ability to tolerate treatments, and other issues, such as financial considerations and your employer's flexibility.

The truth is that you will probably not know how you will react to treatments until after you start them. If possible, you may want to begin with a more limited work schedule (meaning less than what you think you can handle) and then add hours onto your schedule, depending on how you feel and your energy level. Not only will committing to fewer hours prevent you from falling short of expectations at work, but it will also be good for you psychologically. It always feels good to do more than expected (when possible) than to set yourself up for goals that you cannot fulfill. With an altered work schedule, many patients are able to continue working during treatment. If you decide that you cannot work, or if you choose not to work for other reasons during your treatments (such as spending time with your family and friends), you may be eligible for short-term disability through your workplace and/or Social Security Disability (see Question 96).

You will probably not know how you will react to treatments until after you start them.

95. How can I protect myself financially while being faced with expensive treatments for my colorectal cancer?

One of the primary causes of stress among people with cancer is coping with the possible financial issues.

One of the primary causes of stress among people with cancer is coping with the possible financial issues. Financial concerns primarily stem from two sources: the cost of medical care and level of insurance coverage, and the loss of wages caused by temporary or permanent job loss. There are several ways to help reduce the financial impact, including knowing what you can do to protect yourself and learning about possible government and private financial assistance (see Question 96). This topic is complex and varies by geographic region and by individual concerns and situations. Consult your social worker, along with a lawyer or financial planner, to obtain specific information. The following information serves as a guide to help you ask the right questions.

Health Insurance Tips

Contact your health insurance carrier, and if you receive insurance benefits through your employer, contact your human resources department, to discuss your policy coverage as soon as possible. Many insurance companies have established agreements with certain physicians and hospitals, often called the "in-network" medical providers. Furthermore, in order to access this "network" of medical care, a person may first need to be referred by his or her primary care physician. This type of insurance coverage is sometimes referred to as a managed care plan. Different types of insurance plans exist (such as HMOs, POSs, PPOs, etc.), so be sure to contact your provider to get clarification of your coverage. However, it is sometimes possible, even with the most restrictive managed care plans, to receive certain types of cancer treatment out-of-network (from hospitals or doctors who do not have specific agreements with your insurance company), particularly if the treatment is not available by an in-network provider. Be aware that going out-of-network can potentially be more costly to you so make sure that you are fully informed as to the coverage policy where you do decide to get your treatment. Some insurance carriers assign a caseworker if a patient wants to receive treatment out-of-network (or out-of-state), and this person can be a good resource for your insurance-related questions. Be informed of restrictions, such as in--network and out-of-network paperwork, necessary referrals, and/or precertifications. Make sure that you pay all insurance premiums on time. If you do not pay premiums on time, your policy could be terminated, and finding new health coverage with a pre-existing diagnosis can be difficult and expensive.

Document all contact with your human resources department and insurance company, and get everything in writing, such as permission to go out-of-network or referrals to specialists. Include date, time, name of the person with whom you spoke, issues discussed, and resolution or plan. Keep all of this information organized, and always keep copies of any material you send to your insurance company. If you need to dispute coverage decisions, all of this information will be invaluable and will save you time and energy in the long run.

If you think that your insurance company is treating you unfairly, such as denying claims that you believe should be covered or discontinuing your coverage, first contact your insurance company and/or your human resources department. Sometimes simple changes need to be made to fix the problem. For example, claims can be rejected for reasons such as having your incorrect birth date or social security number (SSN) in their computer system or on a form. If an initial inquiry does not work, write a letter to the insurance carrier, clearly stating the claim number, the date of service, your correct personal information (policy and group numbers, SSN, birth date, name, and address), and the reason you believe the claim should have been approved. Be direct but pleasant in your tone, and keep a copy of the letter. The carrier may request additional medical information before covering certain tests or treatments, and sometimes sending additional documentation or having your doctor contact the carrier can resolve these issues. If you have exhausted all options, you can contact your state's insurance commissioner or hire a lawyer who specializes in insurance disputes. Recent legislation at the state and national level exists to protect you, in some limited ways, from insurance coverage lapses due to medical diagnosis and unfair claim rejections. Private insurance companies and health maintenance organizations (HMOs) are most likely regulated by your State Department of Insurance or State Department of Health. See Question 100 for specific references to learn more about these laws and how to seek assistance, including the National Coalition for Cancer Survivorship's publication entitled "What Cancer Survivors Need to Know About Health Insurance."

Work Concerns

If you are currently working or planning to resume work, ask your employer about flexibility in hours to accommodate treatment and appointments, temporary disability insurance, continued health care coverage, and possible leave of absence or family leave. Some people with cancer are fearful of losing their jobs or of being discriminated against because of their diagnosis. Make sure that you are aware of your company's policies and of your legal rights, particularly if you suspect that you are being discriminated against. Legislation, such as the Americans with Disabilities Act (ADA), protects disabled people from certain types of workplace discrimination. A person with cancer or a history of cancer may be protected under the ADA. However, the ADA is complex, applies only to companies that meet specific criteria, and has other limitations. Other federal laws (such as the Federal Rehabilitation Act, the Family and Medical Leave Act, and the Employee Retirement and Income Security Act) and state laws also exist to protect you. Aspects of these laws also pertain to health insurance coverage, particularly The Comprehensive Omnibus Budget Reconciliation Act (COBRA), which makes group insurance policies provided by certain employers available to employees, even those who have quit, been terminated, or work fewer hours. To learn more about work concerns and legislation, consult your social worker or purchase the National Coalition for Cancer Survivorship's publication called "Working It Out: Your Employment Rights As a Cancer Survivor" (see the Appendix for contact information).

96. What government entitlements and benefits can I investigate to help me financially? Are there any private agencies that help colorectal cancer patients with medical expenses?

There are many government programs, particularly at the state and federal level, which can assist with health care coverage and financial assistance for eligible recipients. There are also many other types of private insurance policies, such as long-term care insurance or private disability insurance, and other government programs not discussed here. However, some of the most common programs, along with brief descriptions of each program, are provided below. For more comprehensive information, or for information on programs not mentioned here, speak with your hospital social worker and/or refer to the resources provided in this section and in the Appendix.

Government Programs

Non-means-tested programs (not based on income or assets):

- Medicare (United States Social Security Administration). Federally run health insurance program for people who are either age 65 and over, on Social Security Disability (SSD) (see below) for 2 consecutive years, are legally blind, or on renal dialysis. The information provided here is a brief outline of Medicare coverage; for more information refer to official Medicare web site, www.medicare.gov. Part "A." Usually free to you, but may be purchased if you have not accrued enough Social Security credits based on your work contribution history. Traditionally covers inpatient hospitalization, skilled nursing facility (with specific limitations), **hospice** care, in-home nursing care, and home health care. Deductibles and co-payments may be required. Part "B." Optional, and is purchased by paying monthly premiums (usually $93.50/month in 2007, but may be higher based on income). Covers most medical services, lab tests, outpatient hospital services, medical equipment, supplies (usually including ostomy supplies), and chemotherapy, if administered by your health care provider. Also may cover some preventive care services, including cancer screenings. If you meet Medicaid requirements,the premium may be paid as part of a program called Qualified Medicare Beneficiary Program. Medicare does not typically cover syringes, or insulin for diabetics, experimental treatments, routine medical transportation (ambulance is covered in specific circumstances), or nonmedical or extensive home care services.

Hospice

A type of care focusing on improving quality of life as opposed to extending life when a person is no longer seeking treatment to cure his or her cancer.

- Medicare Managed Care (Medicare Advantage Plans: PPOs, HMOs). Medicare establishes an agreement with certain health insurance companies to manage your insurance coverage. You continue to pay for Part "B" and other fees may be associated with this type of coverage. If you are enrolled in such a program, you may receive added benefits. You will probably be required to choose a primary care physician and may also have added restrictions, such as be limited to in-network medical care, be required to pay additional fees, and more.
- Medicare Part "D" Prescription Drug Coverage. Medicare recently added a prescription coverage component, which may lower drug costs for many people. Typically, the drug coverage benefit is managed by an indepen-

dent insurance company approved by Medicare. This type of coverage usually entails an additional fee, and what exactly is covered can vary across specific plans. All of the specifics of Part "D" are beyond the scope of this brief discussion, For more details contact the Social Security Administration (see the Appendix on page 215 for contact information).

- Medicare Supplemental (or "MediGap" Plans). Purchased by you and is intended to provide additional coverage to people with Medicare, such as prescription drug coverage and other benefits. The government has standardized these plans, and they provide a range of additional coverage. To learn more about these policies, order a copy of The Guide to Health Insurance for People with Medicare (U.S. Department of Health and Human Services; see the Appendix on page 215 for ordering information).
- Social Security Disability (SSD, U.S. Social Security Administration, www.ssa.gov). Provides monthly income to disabled workers and their families based on prior payroll contribution and disabled status. If a person becomes severely disabled before full retirement age, he or she can receive SSD payments after 6 months if he or she has (1) enough social security credits, and (2) a physical or mental impairment that is expected to prevent the person from doing substantial work for 1 year or more, or a condition that is expected to result in death.
- Social Security (SS, U.S. Social Security Administration, www.ssa.gov). Social Security provides monthly payments to persons age 65 and over and family survivors (after the recipient's death, including dependents). Eligibility entails contributing to SS during a person's previous work history, and amount of payment is based on a formula that considers the amount you contributed.

- Veterans' Benefits. If you are a U.S. veteran, contact the Department of Veterans Affairs to investigate benefits for which you are eligible (including possible financial assistance and/or medical care). Qualified veterans can also receive discounts on prescription drugs.

Means-tested (partially or fully based on income and assets) programs:

- Medicaid (State Department of Social Services, http://cms.hhs.gov/medicaid). Medical insurance program for people who live on a limited income. Eligibility and coverage differ from state to state, and some states are more restrictive than others about income limits and eligibility criteria. You may be eligible if you have a low income, have high medical bills, receive Supplemental Security Income (SSI), and/or meet specific other requirements such as citizenship status. Some hospitals can apply for Medicaid while you are a patient. Speak to your hospital's financial services department or social worker to find out more about this. You may also contact your local Medicaid office or Social Services department directly. A directory of state programs is located online at http://cms.hhs.gov/medicaid .
- Medicaid Managed Care. Similar to Medicare Managed Care, some states have allowed Medicaid recipients to enroll in managed care plans. In some states, recipients were automatically enrolled in such programs. However, a person diagnosed with cancer may be able to disenroll from these programs if they find that the managed care policies are too restrictive. Contact your managed care insurance carrier or Medicaid office to investigate the disenrollment process.
- Supplemental Security Income (SSI, U.S. Social Security Administration, www.ssa.gov). Provides monthly income to eligible people over the age of 65, or to blind or disabled people, with low income, few assets, and/or

limited formal work history. May also provide benefits for people waiting for SSD payments to begin. U.S. citizenship is required, with few exceptions. If you are eligible for SSI, then you may also be eligible for Medicaid, food stamps, and other assistance.

- Public Assistance (welfare/food stamps, State Department of Social Services). Provides cash benefits for low-income persons to buy food, clothing, and shelter. Benefits vary depending on assets, income, rent/mortgage, living arrangements, work expenses, and other special needs. Some states require recipients to work, and if they are unable to work due to medical illness, they may require a physician's examination to be exempt. Food stamps provide a monthly allotment of coupons for low-income households to purchase food at grocery stores and meals in some restaurants.

Financial Assistance

Nonprofit agencies and other community resources can sometimes provide limited, temporary assistance for housing, transportation, and other medical expenses not covered by insurance to qualified individuals. Applicants may be required to complete a financial evaluation. Such agencies include Cancer Care, Inc., American Cancer Society, local charities, and your hospital's social work department or financial services department (see the Appendix on page 215 for contact information). However, resources are limited and the availability of funds can change, so you may consider contacting these places directly for information. Some pharmaceutical companies provide limited free or reduced-cost prescriptions to qualified individuals. Often these programs are called "compassionate drug" or "patient assistance" programs. If you are having trouble paying for certain prescriptions, ask your doctor or pharmacist what company makes the drug. Then contact the company to determine whether it has a patient assistance program and how you can apply. You can also try NeedyMeds.com to find information on specific drug or company programs.

97. What is home care, and what can I expect from home care after my surgery and during other treatments?

Home care is a broad term used to describe many types of care services provided in a person's home. Multiple terms used for different types of care are often confusing, so be specific about your wants and needs when you discuss home care options. Medical home care often requires a doctor's order and usually involves a skilled nursing need, such as open wound care, ostomy care, or infusion care. A home health aide (sometimes referred to as a personal care attendant) is a person who is qualified to provide "personal care," such as assisting you with bathing, dressing, and getting around. They most often work for a home health care agency and may also assist with light housework. A home health aide is not usually covered by insurance unless it is ordered in conjunction with a skilled nursing need. A home attendant (or "homemaker" service) is a person who can assist with shopping, house cleaning, doing laundry, cooking, and going with you to appointments, and is usually not covered by most insurance policies.

A common misperception among patients is that they will automatically have insurance-covered home care provided after their discharge from an inpatient admission, particularly after surgery. Insurance companies vary in the specific terms of their coverage, and most cover only skilled needs, usually requiring services to be provided by a registered nurse, a physical therapist, an occupational therapist, or someone with other medical expertise. Coverage sometimes includes a limited number of home health aide hours per week under RN supervision. Patients and family may feel cheated if they were expecting more professional assistance to be covered by insurance. This is an upsetting situation that can be avoided with advance preparation. Contact your insurance carrier and ask about home care coverage and what, exactly, is needed for coverage. You may also ask about durable medical equipment, such as a walker, wheelchair, bedside commode, or hospital bed, before discharge to learn what your insurance covers. Furthermore, it is important for patients and family members to understand the limits of home care, and begin to make arrangements early for caring for the patient at home. This may entail family members helping the recuperating patient after discharge with cooking, cleaning and other needs, and/or providing other types of assistance, such as providing transportation to follow-up doctor visits.

If home care is ordered by your doctor and covered by your insurance, your discharge planning staff member will discuss the type of care you will receive and when the initial home visit will take place. Sometimes the home care agency will contact you directly to establish the details after the official referral has been made. Often a first visit from an intake registered nurse will take place one day to several days after your discharge. He or she will assess your needs and your home to determine the type of care, the frequency of visits, and any equipment/supply needs that you may require. Be sure to accurately describe your diagnosis, surgery, or other treatment side effects, as well as any other concerns or questions you have about managing at home.

Before you leave the hospital, be sure to get the names and numbers of your discharge planner (or whoever you should contact at the hospital if you have problems with the home care that is ordered), the name of the home care agency, and whom you should contact in case of a medical emergency (even after business hours). This information should be located on discharge papers you receive the day you leave the hospital. Patients sometimes leave the hospital without these crucial contact numbers, which can cause added stress if they later have a question. If this information is not given to you, or if you misplace it, ask for it and keep it handy so that you can refer to it when needed.

In addition to medical home care and family or friend caregivers, you may also investigate community agencies that provide various services to a person's home, such as Meals on Wheels (whereby low-cost, prepared meals are delivered directly to your home); senior centers; private nonprofit organizations that serve senior citizens or disabled individuals; volunteer agencies; and churches, synagogues, and other religious centers. If you feel that you cannot manage safely or easily at home, discuss other options with your family and discharge planner, such as private pay home care, nursing home placement, or assisted living options. New LifeStyles (newlifestyles.com) is a good resource for investigating the types of home care, facility placement, and other alternative living arrangements (such as "assisted living").

98. What is a health care proxy and living will?

The death process in Western culture has been dramatically altered in the face of new medical technology that saves and sustains life. With these advancements come difficult decisions on when to use, and withdraw, such treatments. Even with the best care available today, there may come a time when your cancer has progressed beyond conventional treatments. During this time, because of cancer spread to the liver, lungs, or brain, you may not be able to make decisions regarding your own care. Your family members (or another person you designate) will then make medical decisions on your behalf. In order to facilitate the decision-making process and address the communication, emotional, and sometimes ethical issues that arise, a legal system was established, which varies from state to state. The general term used is **advance directive**, which is a legal document placed in your medical record describing your wishes regarding various life-sustaining medical interventions in the event that you cannot communicate your wishes directly. This allows you to take control of your care and preserve your dignity in these complicated situations. To make this less confusing, Caring Connections, a program of the National

Advance directive

Legal documentation that describes your wishes for treatment in the event that you cannot communicate your wishes directly.

Hospice and Palliative Care Organization (NHPCO) provides free information on state-specific advance care planning. (See the Appendix on page 215 for contact information.)

A **living will** describes an individual's wishes regarding specific supportive medical measures toward the end of life and allows you to be very specific regarding individual therapies. The use of prolonged ventilation with a respirator, the placement of tubes for artificial feeding, and the choice for cardiopulmonary resuscitation (CPR) are common topics for clarification in a living will. The information is documented in your patient record and directs the decisions to manage your care should the need arise. For additional clarification, you can assign a **health care proxy** to help make medical decisions if you are too debilitated to do so yourself. A health care proxy (sometimes called a health care agent) is an officially designated medical decision maker, identified verbally or by a legal document, who acts on your behalf if you become temporarily or permanently unable to make medical decisions.

Living will

Document describing an individual's wishes regarding specific supportive medical measures toward the end of life.

Health care proxy

Sometimes called medical durable power of attorney or health care agent; an officially designated medical decision maker (identified by a legal document or verbal identification) authorized to act if you become unable to make medical decisions on your own behalf.

Many states have family consent laws, establishing a clear succession of family members to be identified as a surrogate medical decision maker if you have not otherwise documented your proxy. If you live in such a state, it is important for you to legally identify a health care proxy if you do not want the state-designated family member to be your proxy. For example, the laws usually do not recognize non-married partners (even if you have been together for a long time) as part of the succession. Instead, a parent or adult child, or a more distant relative could be designated as your proxy and make crucial decisions about your care. For this reason, it is often best if your proxy is someone with whom you have a close relationship and who is aware of your feelings about extreme life support measures in the setting of a terminal disease.

In states that do not have family consent laws, such as New York, it is particularly important to have identified a health care proxy and discuss your wishes with that person, since a family member may not have the legal right to make decisions on your behalf without having been formally identified as the health care proxy.

DNR (do not resuscitate) order

Dictates the steps to be taken if a patient is found to be minimally responsive with minimal life signs.

A common component of advance directives and a living will is a **DNR** order, which stands for "do not resuscitate." A DNR order dictates the steps to be taken if a patient is found to be minimally responsive with minimal life signs. It mandates whether medical steps, such as intubation or CPR, should be administered if a patient goes into cardiac arrest. The Patient Self-Determination Act, enacted in 1991, gave all patients the right to accept or refuse resuscitative efforts in accordance with state laws or statutes.

The DNR order is sometimes a difficult issue.

The DNR order is sometimes a difficult issue for patients, families, and health care providers. It is a potentially emotional topic and decision, and may generate conflicts among the people involved if there is disagreement about the right course of action. For example, some patients and family members may believe that, under all circumstances, all efforts should be made to prolong life and would therefore refuse a DNR order. Other people may believe that death should occur more naturally, without life support and other medical interventions, and agree to a DNR order.

Surrogate decision makers who decide to agree to a DNR order may feel guilt that they are giving up, even though they may be acting according to the previously stated wishes of the patient. Physicians may er-roneously feel as though death signifies a personal failure in their medical decision making and judgment. The DNR order is a patient right, however, set up specifically so that patients have the ability to make treatment decisions. All individual feelings and conflicts should be tempered by an understanding of the patient's true wishes. Additionally, it is important to understand that a DNR order does not mean the withdrawal of care. Patients will not be segregated into a separate section of the hospital and neglected;

their medical needs, such as pain control or other medical care, will continue to be provided. The DNR order comes into play only if a patient requires resuscitation.

In addition to protecting yourself with advance directives, initiate a discussion of your wishes with your health care team and your family, particularly your health care proxy—not only so that your wishes are upheld, but also so that your doctor and your proxy understand your wishes. This will help them make decisions. It removes a lot of the burden of making these decisions from your family and friends because they will not have to guess or speculate about your wishes.

99. The doctors say that there is nothing more they can do to treat my cancer, and they have recommended hospice. What do I do now? Just give up?

Kate's Comment:

Even a person in the last days of life is still living and coping with cancer. Hospice care provides pain control and emotional support so that time can be spent with family, good-byes said, and final life work completed. This is not giving up at all but taking the next steps.

This time period is often filled with important decisions. Make sure that you fully understand what the doctor is telling you. He or she may not be able to give you a specific prognosis, but make sure that you are clear about what your doctor is saying about your condition. Why, exactly, is there nothing left to do? If you are interested in getting more treatment, be sure to ask about any other treatments available, including experimental treatments. Remember that you always have the option of seeking another medical opinion.

After investigating your options, you may decide to discontinue treatment, which is sometimes the hardest decision for patients, and physicians, to make. Physicians use different words ("palliation," "supportive care," "compassionate care," and "comfort care") to represent a shift from focusing on curing or lengthening life toward focusing on treating the symptoms of cancer during the later stages of the disease process. Active palliative care sometimes involves chemotherapy, radiation therapy, or surgery to help alleviate such symptoms. This type of care often refers to symptom management, often with the use of medications, and may include hospice care. Additionally, there is a more recent initiative in medical care to blend palliative care during all stages of cancer treatment, from early- to late-stage disease, from initial diagnosis to the dying process. This initiative is to insure that people get the best treatments to cure or treat their cancer but also the best treatments to relieve symptoms negatively impacting people's quality of life.

Medical professionals also may use the word "hospice" and sometimes assume that you know what this means. Hospice is a type of care focusing on improving or maintaining quality of life, as opposed to extending life, when a person is no longer seeking treatment to cure his or her cancer. Hospice can be provided either at home or at an inpatient facility. Hospice focuses on symptom management, meaning alleviating the pain, nausea, and general distress that is common for people during the dying process. Hospices are often staffed by nurses, doctors (who can adjust pain medication), social workers, psychiatrists, chaplains, and other support staff. You may read more about hospice from the resource list in the Appendix (page 215). If you believe the time is right, you may ask your doctor about hospice care if he or she does not initiate this discussion with you.

Hospice focuses on symptom management.

If hospice care is appropriate, and you choose this type of care, hospice services can provide support to you and your caregivers during this phase of your life. Some people are afraid of hospice care, thinking that it means that they have given up hope. Do not think of hospice this way. Furthermore, accepting hospice care will not hasten your death. Conversely, your symptoms will be better managed so that you can spend more quality time with your loved ones and so that you will enjoy the time you do have left as much as possible.

Ending treatment that has not cured the cancer is often a shock for people and family members. For example, you may feel hopeless, overwhelmed, and/or angry (at your doctor for not being able to cure you or at yourself for not "fighting hard enough"). These are all normal reactions. Emotions such as sadness, loss, and despair sometimes follow. Other people may have prepared themselves for when this time was coming and may be more accepting of their inevitable death, particularly if they discussed these issues beforehand with their support system members.

During this time, people in the later stages of the illness often focus on making their last days as positive as possible. If you are in this situation, there are some questions you can ask yourself that may help you understand how you feel and what your wishes are at this time: Do you want to be in the hospital? At home? At a hospice facility? Do you want to be pain free? Who do you want to be with you? What do you want to do before you die? Express your feelings for your loved ones? Make amends with someone? Pray and focus on your spirituality? Do you have any specific religious tasks you want to complete? Do you believe in an afterlife? If so, what do you imagine? Is it fearful or comforting to you?

Answering these questions is difficult. Discussing them with others may be even more difficult. This is a time when many people look back on their lives, focusing on their relationships, the meaning of life and death, and possibly their relationship with God. You may struggle with psychologically understanding and coping with your death. You may also struggle to help your family cope with your death; they may or may not understand your decisions. You may have existential questions not answered, or you may feel anxious about leaving your loved ones. All of these issues and more may arise. Often, meeting with a chaplain, social worker, or your doctor can help find answers to questions and reduce distress about common concerns that arise during the later stages of life.

100. Where can I get more information about colorectal cancer?

It is impossible to discuss all possible aspects of colorectal cancer in one small volume. The Appendix that follows contains organizations, Web sites, and publications that can be useful to colorectal cancer patients and their families.

Appendix

Organizations

American Academy of Medical Acupuncture (AAMA)
4929 Wilshire Boulevard, Suite 428
Los Angeles, CA 90010
(323) 937–5514
www.medicalacupuncture.org
Provides information on what medical acupuncture is and how it can be used to treat certain conditions. The web site includes a list of commonly asked questions and the ability to search for an acupuncturist in your area.

American Cancer Society (ACS)
American Cancer Society National Home Office
1599 Clifton Road N.E.
Atlanta, GA 30329
(800) ACS–2345
(866) 228-4327 TTY
www.cancer.org
ACS is an excellent resource for a wide range of issues, including information on the medical aspects of cancer, coping and family issues, making medical decisions, and much more. In addition to their superb Web site, they also publish a variety of books and pamphlets (see titles in the Pamphlets section of this Appendix), facilitate support groups and lectures run by local ACS offices (you can search the Internet or call for program details), and are involved in advocacy and government policies issues. In some locations, they can provide limited financial assistance to people in financial need who are undergoing treatment for cancer.

Available Pamphlets (a selection, more are available)

"Colorectal Cancer"

"Our Mom Has Cancer"

"American Cancer Society's Health Eating Cookbook, 2nd Edition"

"Caregiving"

"Cancer in the Family"

American Gastroenterological Association
4930 Del Ray Avenue
Bethesda, MD 20814
(301) 654-2055 www.gastro.org
A professional organization for gastroenterologist physician specialists. There is a section, "Patient Center," which contains information about the digestive system, and specifically about digestive conditions, including colorectal cancer.

American Society of Clinical Oncology
1900 Duke Street, Suite 200
Alexandria, VA 22314
(703) 299–0150
www.asco.org
www.peoplelivingwithcancer.org
The American Society of Clinical Oncology primarily comprised of oncology physicians and other professionals. They support education, research, and policy initiatives to improve the prevention, diagnosis, and treatment of cancer. A section of the Web site is dedicated to "People Living with Cancer" (www.peoplelivingwithcancer.org) and provides information on cancer prevention and treatment, and other useful resources, such as specific information on types of oncologists and tips on how to select the best oncologist for you. Also provides specific information on colorectal cancer and information about specific drugs, a medical dictionary, and issues related to coping.

American Society of Colon and Rectal Surgeons
85 W. Algonquin Road, Suite 550
Arlington Heights, IL 60005
(847) 290–9184
www.fascrs.org
The American Society of Colon and Rectal Surgeons is the leading professional society representing more than 1,000 board-certified colon and rectal surgeons dedicated to the treatment of patients with colorectal diseases. Its mission is to assure high quality patient care by advancing the science, prevention, and management of disorders and diseases of the colon, rectum, and anus. The Web site offers information on colon, rectal, and anal disease and can help you find a board-certified colorectal surgeon in your area (go to the Patient Information section).

Association of Cancer Online Resources, Inc. (ACOR)
173 Duane Street, Suite 3A
New York, NY 10013–3334
(212) 226–5525
www.acor.org
ACOR provides information and links to other online resources. One particularly useful feature of the Web site is under the Publications link where you can search for books on specific cancer-related topics (clink on Cancer Bibliography) and other features, such as Medline updates on the latest scientific abstracts about colorectal cancer (clink on The Latest Scientific Abstracts and then choose Colorectal Cancer). http://listserv.acor.org/archives/colon.html is a link to the colon cancer discussion board.

CancerCare, Inc.
275 7th Avenue
New York, NY 10001
(800) 813-HOPE
(212) 712–8400 (administration); (212) 712–8080 (services)
www.cancercare.org
CancerCare is a national nonprofit organization whose mission is to provide free, professional support services to anyone affected by cancer: people with cancer, caregivers, children, loved ones, and the bereaved. CancerCare programs—including counseling, education, financial assistance and practical help—are provided by trained oncology social workers and are completely free of charge. You may find the reliable online information very helpful and may choose to investigate the in-person, online, and telephone support services.

Cancer Hope Network (CHN)
2 North Road, Suite A
Chester, NJ 07930
(877) 879-HOPENET (3638)
(908) 879-4039
www.cancerhopenetwork.org
Cancer Hope Network is a not-for-profit organization that provides free and confidential one-on-one support to cancer patients and their families. We provide that support by matching cancer patients and/or family members with trained volunteers who have themselves undergone and recovered from a similar cancer experience.

Cancer Research and Prevention Foundation of America
1600 Duke Street, Suite 500
Alexandria, VA 22314
(800) 227-2732
(703) 836–4412
Fax: (703) 836–4413
www.crfa.org
Provides information on how to prevent cancer, including colorectal cancer.

CancerSource.com
280 Summer Street, 9th Floor
Boston, Massachusetts 02210-1506
CancerSource.com
The mission of CancerSource.com is to be a comprehensive, accurate, and personalized source of cancer information and services available. The site provides free cancer resources to medical professionals and patients.

CancerWise™/MD Anderson Cancer Center
The University of Texas M. D. Anderson Cancer Center
1515 Holcombe Boulevard
Houston, TX 77030
(800) 392–1611 or (713) 792–6161
Cancerwise.org
CancerWise is a monthly electronic publication that contains information about the latest advancements in cancer treatment and research, support programs and activities, and cancer prevention tips, among other cancer news and information. CancerWise is produced by The University of Texas M. D. Anderson Cancer Center.

Centers for Disease Control and Prevention (CDC)
1600 Clifton Road
Atlanta, GA 30333
(404) 639–3534
(800) 311–3435
www.cdc.gov
www.cdc.gov/cancer/colorctl/index.htm (Colorectal Cancer)
As part of the Department of Health and Human Services, the CDC's mission is to promote health and quality of life by preventing and controlling disease, injury, and disability. You can search for information on a wide-range of medical topics, including cancer-specific issues. Also provides information on the Screen

for Life: National Colorectal Cancer Action Campaign (www.cdc.gov/cancer/screenforlife).

Colon Cancer Alliance (CCA)
1440 Coral Ridge Drive, Suite 386
Coral Springs, FL 33071
(877) 422–2030 (toll free helpline)
www.ccalliance.org
Provides advocacy, information on the medical aspects of colon cancer, and support programs, such as online group support ("CCAChat") and the "CCA Buddies Network" which is a peer-to-peer support system that links survivors with survivors and caregivers with caregivers, for one-on-one support. The Resource Center section of the Web site also has particularly helpful information, including recommended books, helpful organizations, and much more.

The Center for Reproductive Medicine and Infertility
New York Presbyterian Hospital, Weill Medical College of Cornell University
505 East 70th Street, Suite 340
New York, New York 10021
(212) 746.1762
(888) 703.3456
A medical practice in New York City that specializes in treating fertility concerns for men and women wanting to have a baby.

Colorectal Cancer Association of Canada (CCAC)
60 St. Clair Avenue East, Suite 204
Toronto, ON M4T 1N5
Canada
(416) 920-4333
(877) 50-COLON
www.ccac-accc.ca
The Colorectal Cancer Association of Canada (CCAC) is the first nonprofit organization (in Canada) dedicated to supporting people with colorectal cancer, their families, and caregivers. Its mission is to improve the quality of life of patients and increase awareness of the disease. The CCAC organizes public awareness activities and information sessions to help meet the needs and concerns of its members as well as their families and friends. Events to raise awareness are focused on bringing the experience of people living with colorectal cancer to the attention of other patients and their families. The CCAC also

places emphasis on educating the general public about this particular type of cancer.

Colorectal Cancer Network (CCNetwork)
PO Box 182
Kensington, MD 20895
(301) 879-1500
www.colorectal-cancer.net
Provides a list of Web sites and organizations, with general descriptions, all related to the medical and support aspects of coping with colorectal cancer (for both patients and caregivers). Also provides other support services, including chat rooms and support information, and a list of clinical trials related to treatment of colorectal cancer.

Gilda's Club Worldwide
322 Eighth Avenue, Suite 1402
New York, NY 10001
(888) GILDA–4-U
www.gildasclub.org
The mission of Gilda's Club is to provide meeting places where men, women, and children living with cancer and their families and friends can join with others to build emotional and social support as a supplement to medical care. Free of charge and a nonprofit organization, Gilda's Club offers support and networking groups, lectures workshops, and social events in a nonresidential, homelike setting. Named after the comedian, Gilda Radner, who died of cancer. Call or visit the Web site to learn more about the support services the club provides and whether there is a club in your area.

Department of Veterans Affairs
Veterans Health Association
810 Vermont Avenue, NW
Washington, DC 20420
(202) 273–5400 (Washington, DC office)
(800) 827–1000 (local VA office)
www.va.gov
This site provides extensive information for veterans. It is a one-stop site for all concerns regarding veterans health benefits and services. You can download and/or complete eligibility forms online.

FertileHOPE
65 Broadway, Suite 603
New York, NY 10006
www.fertilehope.org
(888) 994-HOPE
Nonprofit organization with the specific focus of providing information about cancer and fertility, such as fertility risks, fertility preservation options, the state of current research, and financial issues.

Harvard Center for Cancer Prevention
Harvard School of Public Health
401 Park Drive, Landmark 3-East
Boston, MA 02215
(617) 998.1034
www.hsph.harvard.edu/cancer/
Information and research on cancer prevention, including printed brochures (information also available on Web site) entitled "You Can Prevent Colorectal Cancer" and "Take Control: Get Tested for Colorectal Cancer," available in multiple languages, and other materials, including Podcasts, on preventing cancer.

America's Health Insurance Plans
601 Pennsylvania Avenue, NW, South Building
Suite 500
Washington, DC 20004
www.hiaa.org
An organization representing the health insurance industry. Publishes guides for consumers and many health insurance-related topics (click on Consumer Information).

Health Resources and Services Administration (HRSA)
Hill-Burton Program
U.S. Department of Health and Human Services
HRSA Information Center
PO Box 2910
Merrifield, VA 22116
(888) ASK-HRSA (275-4772)
www.hrsa.gov
Under the U.S. Department of Health and Human Services, the HRSA Web site provides information on many government initiatives and programs related to providing health care to low-income, isolated, and disadvantaged populations.

LanguageLine Services
1 Lower Ragsdale Drive
Building 2
Monterey, CA 93940
(877) 886-3885
www.languageline.com
The "Personal Interpreter" is a pay-as-you-go service that allows you to access interpreters in more than 140 languages from any phone, 24 hours a day, 7 days a week, 365 days a year. There is a fee to use these services if your hospital does not have a contract with the company; you can use a credit card to pay. The Web site also provides a description of the services provided, including document translation.

National Cancer Institute
NCI Public Inquiries Office
6116 Executive Boulevard
Room 3036A
Bethesda, MD 20892-8322
(800) 4-CANCER/(800) 422-6237)
TTY: (800) 332-8615
www.nci.nih.gov (www.cancer.gov)
Provides extensive information about health-related issues, including information on cancer. The Web site includes information on how to cope with specific treatment side effects, such as pain and fatigue, information on support and coping, and the latest on cancer treatment and prevention. Also includes information on clinical trials and many other topics.

Available Pamphlets (a selection, more are available)

"Colorectal Cancer Screening: Questions and Answers"

"What You Need To Know About Cancer of the Colon and Rectum"

"Chemotherapy and You: A Guide to Self-Help During Treatment"

"Eating Hints for Cancer Patients Before, During, and After Treatment"

"Get Relief From Cancer Pain"

"Helping Yourself During Chemotherapy"

"Pain Control: A Guide for People With Cancer and Their Families"

"Taking Time: Support for People With Cancer and the People Who Care About Them"

"Taking Part in Clinical Trials: What Cancer Patients Need to Know"

"Radiation Therapy and You: A Guide to Self-Help During Cancer Treatment"

Available in Spanish
"Datos sobre el tratamiento de quimioterapia contra el cancer"

"El tratamiento de radioterapia; guia para el paciente durante el tratamiento"

"En que consisten los estudios clinicos? Un folleto para los pacientes de cancer"

National Center for Complementary and Alternative Medicine
NCCAM Clearinghouse
PO Box 7923
Gaithersburg, MD 20898
(888) 644-6226
(301) 519-3153 (international)
TTY: (866) 464-3615 (for hearing impaired)
nccam.nih.gov/
NCCAM is part of the NIH (National Institutes of Health in the U.S. Department of Health and Human Services). This site provides reliable information regarding disease-specific alternative and complementary therapies. The site covers the basics on using these therapies, where to find doctors, research, and clinical trials all related to complementary and alternative medicine.

National Comprehensive Cancer Network
500 Old York Road, Suite 250
Jenkintown, PA 19046
(888) 909-NCCN (6226)
(215) 690-0300
www.nccn.org
This site provides information about leading cancer treatment centers around the United States. It gives specific information regarding those institutions, their specialties, facilities, and resources. The site also provides cancer treatment guidelines specifically written for the patient (approved and cowritten by the American Cancer Society), and a list of resources for patients and families. Go to the Patients tab at the top of the homepage to access this information.

National Coalition for Cancer Survivorship (NCCS)
1010 Wayne Avenue, Suite 770
Silver Spring, MD 20910
(877) NCSS-YES (622-7937)
(301) 650-9127
www.canceradvocacy.org
The National Coalition for Cancer Survivorship is the oldest survivor-led cancer advocacy organization in the country and a highly respected authentic voice at the federal level, advocating for quality cancer care for all Americans and empowering cancer survivors. This organization publishes useful pamphlets and books (see Pamphlets and Books section of this Appendix) on many aspects of managing the medical, financial, and emotional aspects of cancer. You can order, or listen online to, the The Cancer Survival Toolbox (produced in conjunction with the Association of Oncology Social Work and the Oncology Nursing Society).

Available Pamphlets
"Working It Out: Your Employment Rights As a Cancer Survivor"

"What Cancer Survivors Need to Know About Health Insurance"

National Hospice and Palliative Care Organization (NHPCO)
1700 Diagonal Road, Suite 625
Alexandria, VA 22314
(800) 658–8898
(877) 658-8896 (Spanish helpline)
(703) 837-1500
www.nhpco.org
www.caringinfo.org
Provides information on hospice services nationally, including information on communication about hospice, insurance coverage, and locating hospice services. Also, through Caring Connections, information is provided on state-specific advance directive documents.

NeedyMeds.com
NeedyMeds, Inc.
120 Western Avenue
Gloucester, MA 01930

www.needymeds.com
Offers information about programs sponsored by pharmaceutical manufacturers to help people who cannot afford to purchase necessary drugs.

New LifeStyles Online
4144 N. Central Expressway, Suite 1000
Dallas, TX 75204
(800) 820–3013
www.newlifestyles.com
Provides information on independent retirement communities, assisted living, nursing homes, Alzheimer's care, and home or hospice care. You can order a free guide or search online.

Meals on Wheels Association of America
203 S. Union Street
Alexandria, VA 22314
(703) 548-5558
www.mowaa.org
Provides home-delivered meals to those in need, such as people who have trouble grocery shopping or cooking their own food. The Web site allows you to search for local programs.

Social Security Administration (SSA)
Office of Public Inquiries
Windsor Park Building
6401 Security Boulevard
Baltimore, MD 21235
(800) 772-1213, (800)-325-0778 (TTY)
www.ssa.gov
Provides extensive information on Social Security benefits including Social Security Disability (SSD), Medicare, Supplemental Security Income (SSI), contact information for state Medicaid offices, and much more. You may be able to apply online to these programs and even check your claim status.

United Ostomy Association of America (UOAA)
PO Box 66
Fairview, TN 37062-0066
(800) 826-0826
www.uoaa.org

This organization was recently created after the United Ostomy Association ceased operations in September 2005. The UOAA is an association of affiliated, nonprofit, support groups who are committed to the improvement of the quality of life of people who have, or will have, an intestinal or urinary diversion. This organization can connect you to local chapters for information and support, as well as provide general information about ostomies on the Web site or via telephone.

U.S. Department of Health and Human Services (HHS)
200 Independence Avenue
Washington, DC 20201
(202) 619-0257
(877) 696-6775 (toll free)
www.hhs.gov
The mission of this government organization is to protect health and give a special helping hand to those who need assistance. HHS provides information on many topics, including Medicare, Medicaid, childcare and health initiatives, referrals to information on cancer, and much more.

Available Pamphlet

"Guide to Health Insurance for People with Medicare"

Post-Treatment Resource Program
Memorial Sloan-Kettering Cancer Center
215 E 68th Street, Ground Floor
New York, NY 10021
(212) 717-3527
http://www.mskcc.org/mskcc/html/19409.cfm
Focuses on facilitating support groups, educational lectures, and other support services to people who have completed their cancer treatment.

The Wellness Community
National Office
919 18th Street, NW, Suite 54
Washington, DC 20006
(888) 793-WELL (9355)
(202) 659-9709
www.thewellnesscommunity.org
Provides supportive services to people with cancer and their loved ones by providing a variety of services, including online information and support

(through the Virtual Wellness Community) on-site at locations nationwide (and internationally in Japan and Israel). Also includes a list of suggested books addressing common issues people with cancer and their families face.

Available Pamphlet

"Frankly Speaking About New Discoveries in Cancer: Special Focus on Colorectal Cancer"

Web Sites on Specific Topics

Alternative Therapies

American Academy for Medical Acupuncture (AAMA)

Includes information on acupuncture and allows you to search for local medical acupuncturists.
www.medicalacupuncture.org

National Center for Complementary and Alternative Medicine (NCCAM)

www.nccam.nih.gov

National Cancer Institute

Complementary and Alternative Medicine
http://www.cancer.gov/cancertopics/treatment/cam

Chemotherapy

You Are Not Alone

www.yana.org
Offers online and in-person support groups for those going through high-dose chemotherapy. Groups currently are offered in California, but other in-person groups are starting in other areas of the United States.

National Cancer Institute

NCI Drug Dictionary
www.cancer.gov/drugdictionary/
Self-help information
www.cancer.gov/cancertopics/treatment/types-of-treatment

Clinical Trials

National Cancer Institute
www.cancer.gov/clinicaltrials
CancerTrials site lists current clinical trials that have been reviewed by NCI.

American Cancer Society
Clinical trials information
http://www.cancer.org/docroot/ETO/ETO_6.asp

Survivorship

National Coalition for Cancer Survivorship
www.canceradvocacy.org
Offers a free audio program (also available to listen to online)—"Cancer Survivor Toolbox"—including ways to cope with the illness. Web site also has a newsletter, requiring a yearly membership fee.

Ostomy/Stoma Information

United Ostomy Association of America, Inc.
www.uoaa.org
Provides support and information regarding ostomy care, including support and educational groups, newsletters, online information, and more.

Diet and Nutrition (Cancer Prevention)

USDA Dietary Guidelines
www.usda.gov/cnpp

American Institute for Cancer Research
www.aicr.org
Tips on how to reduce cancer risk.

Genetic Counseling

The National Society of Genetic Counselors
www.nsgc.org

The National Cancer Institute
http://cancer.gov/cancerinfo/prevention-genetics-causes/genetics
Has a searchable list of health care professionals who specialize in genetics and can provide information and counseling.

Legal Protections, Financial Resources, and Insurance Coverage

The American Cancer Society
www.cancer.org
Search using keyword "insurance." Provides information to help you understand your coverage and legal protections, in addition to how to find possible financial assistance.

Centers for Medicaid and Medicare Services
www.cms.hhs.gov
Provides extensive information and referral information on Medicaid and Medicare, including information on individual state plans and how to apply.

National Coalition for Cancer Survivorship
www.canceradvocacy.org
"Working It Out: Your Employment Rights As a Cancer Survivor"
"What Cancer Survivors Need to Know About Health Insurance"

Treatment Locators: Physicians and Hospitals

AIM DocFinder (State Medical Board Executive Directors)
www.docboard.org
Nonprofit organization providing a health professional licensing database.

AMA Physician Select (American Medical Association)
webapps.ama-assn.org/doctorfinder/home.html
AMA database of demographic and professional information on individual physicians in the United States.

American Board of Medical Specialties
www.abms.org
(866) ASK-ABMS
Provides verification of physician qualifications and has lists of specialists.

Best Hospitals Finder (U.S. News & World Report)
www.usnews.com/usnews/health/best-hospitals/hosp_search.htm
The U.S. News & World Report hospital rankings are designed to assist patients in their search for the highest level of medical care. Database is searchable by specialty, including the top cancer hospitals.

National Cancer Institute Designated Cancer Centers
www.cancer.gov/clinicaltrials/finding/NCI-cancer-centers/map
Directory of NCI-designated Cancer Centers, 58 research-oriented U.S. institutions recognized for scientific excellence and extensive cancer resources. Listings feature phone contact numbers, Web site links, and a brief summary of Web site resources.

Approved Hospital Cancer Program
Commission on Cancer of the American College of Surgeons
www.facs.org/cancer/index.html
The Approvals Program of the Commission on Cancer surveys hospitals, treatment centers, and other facilities according to standards set by the Committee on Approvals, which recommends approval awards in specific categories based on these surveys. A hospital that has received approval has voluntarily committed itself to providing the best in diagnosis and treatment of cancer. Approved hospitals can be searched by city, state, and category.

Physician Qualifications

The American Board of Medical Specialties
www.abms.org
Click on Who's Certified button and search by physician name or by specialty.

Books

100 Questions and Answers about Caring for Family or Friends with Cancer by Rose, Susannah & Hara, Richard, Jones and Bartlett Publishers, 2005.

How to Help Children Through a Parent's Serious Illness by Kathleen McCue, St. Martin's Griffin, 1994.

A Cancer Survivor's Almanac: Charting Your Journey, Second Edition by Barbara Hoffman, JD (Ed), National Coalition for Cancer Survivorship, John Wiley & Sons, 1998.

The Human Side of Cancer: Living With Hope, Coping With Uncertainty by Jimmie Holland, MD and Sheldon Lewis, HarperCollins, San Francisco, 2000.

Informed Decision: The Complete Book of Cancer Diagnosis, Treatment, and Recovery, Second Edidtion by Harmon Eyre, Dianne Lange, and Lois Morris, American Cancer Society, 2001.
Available at by the American Cancer Society for purchase.

Beyond Miracles: Living with Cancer: Inspirational and Practical Advice for Patients and Their Families by Stephen Hersh, Seven Locks Press, 2000.

When a Parent Has Cancer: A Guide to Caring for Your Children by Wendy S. Harpham, HarperCollins, 2004.

Facing Cancer Together: How to Help Your Friend or Loved One, by Pamela Brown with Dave Dravecky, Augsburg Fortress Publishers, 1999.

When Life Becomes Precious: The Essential Guide for Patients, Loved Ones, and Friends of Those Facing Serious Illnesses by Elise Babcock, Bantam, 1997.

Handbook for Mortals: Guidance for People Facing Serious Illness by Joanne Lynn and Joan Harrold, Oxford University Press, 2001.

Glossary

A

Abdominoperineal resection (APR): Surgical removal of the anus, the rectum, and the surrounding muscles of the anal canal. Because the muscles of the anal sphincter are removed, a permanent colostomy is required.

Acupuncture: A Chinese therapy involving the use of thin needles placed in special pressure points on the body.

Adenocarcinoma: Cancerous tumor arising from glandular cells.

Adenoma: Glandular tumor arising from the mucosa of the colon. It is a benign (noncancerous) lesion that is confined to the mucosa. Adenomas are premalignant lesions and over time can degenerate into an invasive tumor.

Adenoma-carcinoma sequence: The process by which a benign adenoma is transformed into cancer.

Adjuvant therapy: Nonsurgical treatment option for cancer that helps improve long-term survival.

Advance directive: Legal documentation that describes your wishes for treatment in the event that you cannot communicate your wishes directly.

Amsterdam criteria: Screening guidelines used to identify families with hereditary nonpolyposis colon cancer (HNPCC).

Anal canal: The end of the gastrointestinal tract where the rectum is surrounded by the muscles of the anal sphincter.

Anal sphincter: Muscular band that allows us to maintain fecal continence.

Anastomosis: Surgical connection between ends of bowel.

Anemia: Decreased number of red blood cells.

Angina: Chest pain that results from atherosclerotic heart disease.

Anterior resection: Surgical removal of the lower portion of the sigmoid colon or upper rectum that is performed through an incision in the lower abdomen.

Antibody: Molecule in the body's immune system that identifies foreign substances on bacteria and cancer cells.

Anticoagulant: Medication that inhibits normal blood clotting.

Antihypertensive: Medication used to lower blood pressure.

Aorta: The major arterial blood vessel arising from the heart.

Artery: Any blood vessel that carries blood (usually oxygenated) away from the heart to other organs.

B

Barium enema: An x-ray examination of the colon using a contrast material to highlight the area being examined.

Benign: A tumor that lacks the ability to invade or spread.

Bilary Sclerosis: Bile duct scarring.

Biopsy: A procedure in which tissue is removed and examined.

Bolus: A dose of drug given intravenously all at once, rather than by slow infusion.

Bowel: another word for intestine.

Brachytherapy: Radiation therapy consisting of the surgical placement of small catheters (hollow tubes) into the body. The catheters administer the radiation either into or adjacent to where the cancer was situated.

C

Cancer: The disordered and uncontrolled growth of cells.

Carcinogenic: Able to induce cancer.

Carcinoid tumor: Tumor consisting of neuroendocrine (hormone producing) cells.

Carcinoma in situ: Malignant cells that are confined to the colonic or rectal mucosa but do not invade the underlying submucosa. This is the earliest stage of pre-colon cancer. These tumors cannot spread to distant sites.

Catheter: A hollow tube used to drain or inject fluid.

CEA (carcinoembryonic antigen) level: A test to detect a protein that is often created by colon cancers. Used primarily as a surveillance test for recurrent colorectal cancer.

Cecum: The pouch-like structure that is the first segment of the colon.

Cell: The smallest structural unit of a living organism.

Chemoradiation: Therapy consisting of chemotherapy and radiation therapy.

Chemotherapy: The use of drugs to treat disease; in this case, cancer.

Chromosomes: thread-like structures inside the nucleus of the cell that contain the genetic instructions for cell function.

Colectomy: Surgical removal of all or part of the colon.

Colitis: Inflammation of the colon.

Colon: Part of the large intestine beginning at the cecum and continuing until the end of the sigmoid colon where the rectum begins.

Colonoscopy: Video-endoscopy of the entire colon.

Colorectal surgeons: Physicians who specialize in surgery for benign and malignant disorders of the colon and rectum; they also perform endoscopy of the lower GI tract.

Colostomy: Stoma (a loop of bowel brought surgically out through the abdominal wall) created using the colon.

Complementary therapy: A new treatment intended to be used in addition to the standard proven treatment option.

Computed tomography (CT): Radiologic examination that utilizes x-rays to generate a two-dimensional computer image of the area scanned. In people diagnosed with colorectal cancer, CT scanning is used primarily to evaluate the liver for metastatic spread.

Corticosteroids: Immune-modulating medications used in the treatment of inflammatory bowel disease.

Crohn's disease: An inflammatory bowel disease that can affect any part of the gastrointestinal tract. Crohn's disease of the colon is characterized by an inflammatory process that extends through the entire bowel wall and can cause strictures (narrowings) and fistulas (abnormal connections between two organs).

Cryoablation: An invasive technique that destroys tumor cells through the freezing and thawing of malignant tissue.

D

Defecation: The act of moving one's bowels.

Diverticulitis: Inflammation of a diverticulum.

Diverticulosis: Multiple diverticula within the colon. They are most commonly found in the sigmoid colon.

Diverticulum: Abnormal out-pouching of mucosa through the colonic wall.

DNA (deoxyribonucleic acid): The building block of chromosomes.

DNR (do not resuscitate) order: Dictates the steps to be taken if a patient is found to be minimally responsive with minimal life signs. It mandates whether medical steps, like intubation or CPR, should be administered.

Dysplasia: Microscopic finding of abnormal cellular growth characterized by overcrowding of cells and irregularly shaped nuclei.

E

Electric cautery or electrocautery: Using electricity to destroy tissue.

Endometrium: The lining inside the uterus.

Endorectal ultrasound: Radiographic test using refracted sound waves to evaluate local tumor spread within the rectum.

Endoscope: A lighted instrument used to look inside a body cavity.

Endoscopy: Using a lighted instrument to look inside a body cavity

Enterostomal specialist: Usually a nurse with special training in ostomy care, including coping with body changes after surgery.

Epidermis: Outermost layer of the skin.

Epidural anesthesia: Anesthesia that is administered via a small catheter that is inserted into the epidural space around the spinal cord.

Esophagus: Muscular tube joining the mouth and stomach.

Excision: Surgical removal.

External-beam radiation therapy: Radiation therapy delivered through the skin.

F

FAP (familial adenomatous polyposis): Disease characterized by the development of multiple adenomatous polyps throughout the colon, usually at a young age.

Fecal occult blood testing (FOBT): Laboratory test that examines stool for microscopic traces of blood.

Fistula: Abnormal connection between two hollow organs.

Food and Drug Administration (FDA): The government agency responsible for the approval of medications and new therapies in the United States.

G

Gardner's syndrome: A variant of familial adenomatous polyposis that is associated with bone tumors, polyps, and abdominal tumors.

Gastric: related to the stomach.

Gastroenterologist: medical doctor who specializes in disorders of the gastrointestinal tract.

Gastrointestinal (GI) tract: group of organs involved in the digestion and absorption of the food we eat.

Gene: a segment of DNA within a chromosome that contains the information to create a single protein.

Germline mutations: errors in the genetic code that are transferred between family members.

Grade: measure of a tumor's size.

H

Health care proxy: sometimes called medical durable power of attorney or health care agent; an officially designated medical decision maker (identified by a legal document or verbal identification) authorized to act if you become unable to make medical decisions on your own behalf.

Hemoglobin: protein in the blood responsible for carrying oxygen.

Hepatic: relating to the liver.

Hepatic artery infusion (HAI): a technique that uses a pump to administer high doses of chemotherapy directly into the blood supply of the liver.

Hereditary nonpolyposis colon cancer (HNPCC): syndrome of inherited colon cancer and other associated cancers that is not associated with the familial adenomatous polyposis syndrome. Often referred to as the Lynch syndrome.

Hernia: a loop of bowel or an organ that protrudes through an abnormal opening in the body.

Histologic: microscopic appearance.

Hormones: chemical messengers passed through the blood stream that affect other organs.

Hospice: a type of care focusing on improving quality of life as opposed to extending life when a person is no longer seeking treatment to cure his or her cancer.

Hyperproliferation: abnormally high rate of cell division and reproduction.

Hypertension: high blood pressure.

Hypnosis or hypnotherapy: a type of therapy, led by a trained professional, that helps people focus on a specific issue or sensation with the intention of treating a certain problem, such as pain or stress. People can also learn how to hypnotize themselves.

I

Ileocecal valve: junction of the small and large intestine.

Ileostomy: stoma created with small bowel.

Ileus: delayed bowel function after abdominal surgery.

Impotence: inability to maintain an erection that is sufficient to engage in sexual activity.

Imuran: drug that suppresses the body's immune system. Imuran is utilized in the treatment of inflammatory bowel disease.

Incidence: the number of new cases of a disease over a given time period, usually over 1 year.

Insufflation: the blowing of air into a body cavity.

Insulin: hormone responsible for stabilizing blood sugar.

Interstitial fluid: contains absorbed nutrients and cellular waste products that are recycled back into the bloodstream to be metabolized and detoxified.

Intravenously: medications given through the veins.

Ischemia: insufficient blood flow resulting in inadequate tissue oxygenation.

J

Jaundice: the symptoms that are associated with liver failure; especially a yellow color to your skin and the whites of your eyes.

L

Large intestine (colon and rectum): the final organ in the gastrointestinal tract. Its role is the absorption of water and nutrients from digested waste.

Living will: document describing an individual's wishes regarding specific supportive medical measures toward the end of life.

Low anterior resection: resection of the lower rectum through a lower midline abdominal incision.

Lumen: the area inside a hollow organ.

Lymph nodes: small pea-like structures that strain the interstitial fluid of bacteria, toxins, and cancer.

M

Magnetic Resonance Imaging (MRI): a diagnostic radiology study that uses nuclear technology, including radiofrequency signals and a strong magnetic field, to provide 3-D images of the body's interior, delineating muscle, bone, blood vessels, nerves, organs, and tumor tissue. Unlike conventional radiography or CT scanning, MRI does not expose patients to ionizing radiation.

Malignant: a tumor that can invade and spread.

MediPort (Port-a-Cath): permanent central venous catheter that is placed underneath the skin and usually used for long-term chemotherapy.

Mesenteric vessels: the blood vessels that supply the large and small intestine. The lymph channels that drain the colon and rectum are adjacent to these vessels.

Mesentery: the fatty tissue surrounding the blood vessels that supply the bowel.

Metastases: the distant spread of a cancer from its organ of origin.

Mortality: the death rate from a specific disorder.

MRI: see magnetic resonance imaging.

Mucosa: the moist membrane lining the inside of the colon containing small glands that secrete mucus.

Muscularis: the muscle layer of the bowel wall.

Mutation: a genetic error.

Myocardial infarction: damage to heart cells as a result of decreased blood flow; a heart attack.

N

Nasogastric (NG) tube: suction tube placed through the nose down into the esophagus and stomach to drain gastric contents.

Neoadjuvant therapy: radiation therapy and chemotherapy given before surgery.

Neoplasm: abnormal growth of cells, a tumor.

Neuropathy: disruption in a nerve's function, sometimes caused by trauma, such as during surgery.

Nonsteroidal anti-inflammatory drug (NSAID): category of drugs that reduce inflammation; includes aspirin, ibuprofen, sulindac.

O

Occult: hidden; not obvious to the naked eye.

Ostomy: a surgically created opening from the inside to the outside of the body.

P

Palliative therapy: noncurative therapy with the aim of making the patient more comfortable.

Pancolitis: colitis involving the entire colon.

Pathology: the branch of science that studies the nature of disease processes.

Patient-controlled analgesia (PCA): pump connected to an intravenous line that allows pain medication to be self-administered by a patient.

Pedunculated polyp: a polyp growing on a stalk.

Percutaneously: through the skin.

Perineum: the area of the body around the anus and genital structures.

Peritoneal cavity: abdominal cavity.

Platelets: blood cells responsible for blood clotting.

Polyp: abnormal mucosal growth.

Polypectomy: surgical removal of polyps.

Polyposis: condition in which multiple polyps form in an organ.

Positive coping: a term the author uses to refer to a person's unique methods of managing distress, including focusing on a positive attitude, in addition to identifying and addressing the negative reactions to having cancer.

Positron emission tomography (PET): radiographic study that uses the abnormal sugar metabolism of cancer cells to identify metastatic deposits.

Preadmission testing: workup before your surgery that includes screening blood tests, electrocardiogram, and chest x-ray.

Precancer: abnormal cells that do not yet have the capacity to spread.

Proctectomy: surgical removal of the rectum.

Proctocolectomy: surgical removal of colon and rectum.

Proctoscopy: evaluation of the rectum using a rigid or flexible endoscope.

Prognosis: the predicted course of the disease.

Progressive relaxation: a method of stress reduction in which a person can focus on breathing and on relaxing body parts individually to gradually become more relaxed and less stressed.

Prophylactic: for the purpose of prevention.

R

Radiation therapy: the use of high-energy electromagnetic radiation to treat cancer by damaging cell DNA and causing cell death.

Radical surgery: surgery designed to remove diseased areas and also areas that might have been affected by the disease.

Radiofrequency ablation: cancer treatment that uses heat to kill tumors.

Rectum: pouch-like structure within the lower part of the large intestine that stores fecal waste before defecation.

Restorative proctocolectomy: a surgical procedure in which the entire colon and rectum are removed, but a rectum is created using a pouch constructed from small bowel (J-pouch).

Retrograde ejaculation: the flow of semen backwards into the bladder rather than out through the penis.

S

Salvage resection: surgical removal of a cancer after less radical initial treatments have failed.

Sarcoma: a stromal cancer that is highly likely to spread.

Sensitivity: the ability of a screening test to identify patients with the disease.

Serosa: thin external lining of the bowel surface.

Sessile polyp: a flat-appearing polyp.

Sigmoid colon: the "S"-shaped loop of colon before the rectum.

Sigmoidoscopy: examination of the rectum and sigmoid colon by an endoscope.

Simulation: the initial consultation with your radiation oncologist where the exact fields for your radiation will be created.

Small intestine: tubular organ between the stomach and the large intestine. The function of the small intestine is the breakdown and absorption of the food we eat. Also called the small bowel.

Sphincter (anal sphincter): circular muscle around the anus that enables us to hold waste inside.

Sphincter-saving surgery: surgery for removal of a rectal cancer that is able to spare the sphincter muscles and therefore avoid a permanent colostomy.

Sporadic mutation: a genetic error that occurs randomly and is not an inherited flaw.

Squamous cell carcinoma (SCC): cancer arising from the lining of the anal canal.

Stage: a characterization of the extent of tumor growth and spread.

Stoma: a loop of bowel brought surgically out through the abdominal wall.

Stricture: narrowing of the lumen of bowel because of scarring, inflammation, or tumor.

Stomach: the sac-shaped digestive organ that is located in the upper abdomen, under the ribs.

Stromal tumor: rare tumor that starts in the muscular layers of the colon.

Submucosa: the layer of the bowel wall between the glandular lining (mucosa) and the muscle layer.

Sulindac: a nonsteroidal anti-inflammatory drug that may help prevent formation of colonic polyps.

T

Therapeutic ratio: the dose required to treat the cancer divided by the tolerance dose of the surrounding organs.

Total mesorectal excision (TME): surgical removal of most of the rectum and its entire mesentery.

Transanal excision (TAE): sphincter-saving technique for removal of small tumors of the lower rectum. During transanal excision, an abdominal incision is avoided, and the tumor is removed through the anus.

Transcription: the conversion of DNA into its messenger RNA.

Tumor: abnormal growth of tissue.

Turcot's syndrome: variant of familial adenomatous polyposis that is associated with brain tumors.

U

Ulcerative colitis: inflammatory disease affecting the mucosa of the large intestine. Individuals with ulcerative colitis have a higher risk of developing colorectal cancer.

Umbilicus: belly button.

Urologist: surgeon who specializes in diseases of the urinary tract.

Index

Page numbers in italics indicate figures or tables.